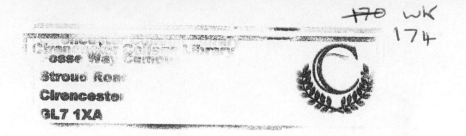
Moral Problems in Medicine
A Practical Coursebook

Moral Problems
in Medicine

A Practical Coursebook

Michael Palmer

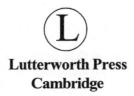

Lutterworth Press
Cambridge

The Lutterworth Press
P. O. Box 60
Cambridge
CB1 2NT

e-mail: publishing@lutterworth.com
Web site: http://www.lutterworth.com

British Library Cataloguing in Publication Data:
A catalogue record is available from the British Library

ISBN 0 7188 2978 6

Printed in Great Britain by
MPG Books Ltd, Bodmin, Cornwall

IN MEMORY OF MY GODSON
JOE HARKNESS
28.iii.1980 – 28.xi.1997

Contents

Introduction

This book is primarily intended for those interested in seeing how certain philosophical arguments can impinge directly on specific moral problems in medicine. It is first and foremost a book *for the beginner* in as much as it requires no previous knowledge of philosophy and indeed no prior understanding of the kind of moral issues that arise in the practice of medicine. That said, I am well aware that many of my readers, if a little hazy about philosophy, will be much less so about medicine; and that many of them – I am thinking here in particular of those with special interests in applied ethics, for example, health care professionals and social workers – will already have had quite direct experience of many of the issues I raise. For them, I hope, this book will provide some insight into how philosophy can be of use.

Because this book incorporates material that has been published already in a work of mine, I should first say something about that earlier publication. In 1991 Lutterworth Press published my *Moral Problems.* As is usual with books of this type, my publishers and I looked forward to steady if unspectacular sales over a limited period of time. That this has not been the case came, therefore, as a delightful surprise to us both. But perhaps, on reflection, we should have been more optimistic about the book's prospects. Philosophy is no longer viewed as a subject confined to universities, and the last few years have witnessed a remarkable expansion in the teaching of philosophy at other levels. In the United Kingdom, for example, there are now national examinations in the subject and it figures prominently in other associated examinations such as religious studies, politics, and general studies. At a non-examinable level, it is equally refreshing to see how more and more schools and colleges, in the quest to broaden their curricula, have introduced a philosophical component into many of their courses. In the United States, the development of philosophy has been equally dramatic, not only in high schools and colleges but, more famously, with the introduction of philosophy courses specially designed for eight- and nine-year-olds. Another feature of this expansion, on both sides of the Atlantic, has been the increasing use of philosophy in the training of those entering particular professions, such as the law, business, and medicine.

Moral Problems covered a wide variety of topics. Quite apart from the analysis of major ethical theories, it included sections on moral issues as diverse as civil disobedience, abortion, euthanasia, crime and punishment, warfare, and many others. This new book, while retaining the philosophical component of the earlier one, now restricts the discussion solely to medical matters, thereby allowing for a greater range and depth within that area. This has allowed me, for example, to extend the treatment of abortion and euthanasia, and to add other relevant topics such as those to do with medical experimentation, lying to patients, confidentiality, and genetic technology, to name a few.

Moral Problems in Medicine retains other features borrowed from *Moral*

Problems. The first to mention is that, like its predecessor, this book is not a compendium of ethical thought, any more than it is a handbook detailing all the possible dilemmas that a doctor or nurse might face in their working lives – if indeed such a thing were possible. It is primarily a *course book,* providing the instructor, student, and interested reader with a step-by-step introduction to ethical theory, with each theory being thereafter illustrated and applied in a specific medical context. This has imposed on me certain inevitable restrictions. Most obviously, lack of space has meant that I have had to be selective in the theories and issues that I discuss, and I am all too well aware that there are many omissions, which many may object to. I realise that for those already familiar with the philosophical literature the absence of, for example, existentialist or Marxist or Christian ethics will be a serious one. The same holds true for those acquainted with the medical literature, and they too may be surprised that I pay scant attention to such matters as foetal research, organ donation, the allocation of limited medical resources, care of the elderly, resuscitation orders, and many other matters of moral concern, all of which often feature in medical textbooks. But here I can only reply that completeness has not been my first priority. My primary ambition has been to promote some understanding of how medical decisions incorporate ethical viewpoints, and for this, it seems to me, an encyclopaedic approach is not always helpful. What one requires here is the detail but not necessarily the scope.

This concern to relate, as closely as possible, the ethical theory to a particular medical issue also explains the sequence of chapters and the so-called Discussion sections of the course. In these sections my concern has been to show how the ethical theory operates within a particular medical-ethical dilemma. So the chapter on utilitarianism is followed by a discussion-chapter on experimentation, the chapter on Kant by another dealing with the question of whether doctors should tell their patients the truth about their condition, and so on. An introduction to each medical issue is provided, and the issue itself presented by three short extracts from original sources.

This use of original texts is another priority I have retained from *Moral Problems.* Not only has it always seemed strange to me that someone can become familiar with, say, utilitarianism, without ever having read Bentham, but it seems equally important to me, in the medical context, to read accounts both from those who are specialists in their field and from those who write from first hand experience of the practical implications of a medical decision. A case in point is the famous article by Dr Timothy Quill, included in this volume, which raises the question of whether doctors should assist in the suicide of terminally ill patients.

My final priority has been to furnish readers with as much help as possible in what may be, after all, unfamiliar territory. Throughout the book I have therefore included various exercises at points in the text where I think some clarification helpful. All chapters include a number of essay questions and a bibliography.

The structure of the book may therefore be summarised as follows:

THE ETHICAL THEORY
Introduction
Original Text
Exercises
Criticism
Essay Questions
Bibliography

DISCUSSION: A MORAL PROBLEM IN MEDICINE
Introduction
Original Texts
Essay Questions
Bibliography

As a final word, I should like to express my thanks to Lutterworth Press, with which I have now been happily associated for many years; and in particular to its Managing Director, Adrian Brink, who first raised the possibility of presenting an earlier work of mine in this new form.

Michael Palmer

Chapter 1
Ethics

1. WHAT IS ETHICS?

All of us, at some time or other, are faced with the problem of what we ought to do. It is not difficult to think of examples. We accept that we ought to help a blind person cross the road or that we ought to tell the truth in a court of law. We also recognise that we ought not to cheat in examinations and ought not to drink and drive. These 'oughts' and 'ought nots' are clear to us, although this does not necessarily mean that we always act accordingly. Because of this we also attach praise and blame to our own actions and those of others.

In all these cases we are making **moral** or **ethical** judgements. In these judgements we decide that this action is right or wrong or that person is good or bad. Ethics is, therefore, usually confined to the area of human character or conduct, the word 'ethics' deriving from the Greek *ethikos* (that which relates to *ethos* or character.) Men and women generally describe their own conduct and character, and that of others, by such general terms as 'good', 'bad', 'right' and 'wrong'; and it is the meaning and scope of these adjectives, in relation to human conduct, that the moral philosopher investigates. The philosopher is not, however, concerned with merely a *descriptive* account of the attitudes and values that people hold: that 'X believes that war is wrong' or that 'Y believes that abortion is right'. That X and Y believe these things may be of interest to the anthropologist or sociologist, but they are of little interest to moral philosophers. What concerns them is not *that* X and Y should believe these things but *why* they do. Ethics, in other words, is much more than explaining what you or I might say about a particular moral problem; it is a study of the reasoning behind our moral beliefs, of the *justification* for the particular moral positions we adopt.

The study of ethics is split into two branches. First, there is **normative ethics**. Here we consider what kinds of things are good and bad and how we are to decide what kinds of action are right and wrong. This is the main tradition of ethical thinking, extending back to Socrates, Plato and Aristotle, and the one we are most concerned with in this book.

Then there is **meta-ethics**, a detailed account of which is given in the Appendix. Meta-ethics deals with a philosophical analysis of the meaning and character of ethical language; with, for example, the meaning of the terms 'good' and 'bad', 'right' and 'wrong'. Meta-ethics is, therefore, *about* normative ethics and seeks to understand the terms and concepts employed there. For example, when I say 'Saving life is good' I might well begin a normative debate about when I should and should not do such a thing. Do I mean that all lives should be saved or only some? But in meta-ethics, I will be concerned much more with the meaning of the term 'good' within the sentence 'Saving life is good'. Is it something I can find in objects, so that I can easily detect it in some and not in others? Or is it something I can see (like a colour) or something I can feel (like a toothache)? In recent years, largely through philosophy's increasing preoccupation with the analysis of language, this branch of ethics has tended to dominate ethical discussion. It is held that one cannot even begin normative ethics without a prior analysis of the terms being used. Certainly the overlap between the two is extensive, although whether meta-ethics is necessarily prior to normative ethics is an open question and the subject of considerable philosophical dispute.

From what has been said so far, it may be gathered that ethical statements are statements of a particular kind. They are not, for example, straightforward *empirical* statements, i.e. statements of demonstrable fact. If we say 'Atomic weapons kill people', we are stating a simple observable fact; but if we say 'Atomic weapons should be banned', we are stating what we believe ought to happen. In the first case, it is easy to establish whether the statement is true or false; but in the second, this is clearly impossible. In this instance, we are not stating facts so much as giving a value to certain facts – and a negative value at that. We are expressing a point of view about a particular circumstance, which we also know is not shared by everyone. This is not to say that all propositions that give value to something are ethical propositions. We might say that 'Rolls-Royce make good cars' or 'That is a bad tyre', but we would not be attributing moral value to the cars or tyre. Similarly, in the area of art judgements (or aesthetics), we might speak of a 'good painting' or 'bad play', but usually we are not referring to the moral significance of the painting or play. All these, then, are non-moral uses of the words 'good' and 'bad'.

Exercise 1

How is the term 'good' being used in the following sentences? Which of these sentences are morally or ethically significant?

a.   That music is good
b.   Democracy is a good thing
c.   He is a good footballer
d.   He did me no good
e.   This is a good report
f.   He had a good life
g.   He led a good life
h.   It is good to tell the truth
i.   Did you have a good holiday?
j.   Take a good look
k.   He has good manners
l.   It is good to see you
m.   God is good

2. WHAT IS MEDICAL ETHICS?

Medical ethics covers those questions about what ought and ought not to be done in a defined area of human activity: the practice of medicine. These questions may well involve a wide range of people – not just the doctor but the nurse, patient, relative and, beyond them, members of the community – and are invariably raised in situations of extreme moral stress, where, often for the first time, individuals are involved in decisions of life and death. In recent years, however, interest in medical ethics has grown quite remarkably. There seems to be two reasons for this. 1) The first has to do with the tremendous scientific and technological advances that have taken place in medicine during the latter half of this century, and which have given physicians and other health-care professionals the ability to keep patients alive in circumstances where they would previously have died. We can now resuscitate those whose cardiopulmonary functioning has ceased; we can transplant kidneys, livers and hearts; we can provide artificial implants such as cardiac pacemakers, arterial grafts and intra-ocular lenses, and so on. 2) These recent developments in medical technology have highlighted, as never before, some particular moral dilemmas. Should, for example, these techniques of sustaining life be always applied? Should a patient's life be preserved in all cases or might there be cases in which the patient should be allowed to die? And who is to decide between these cases? All these questions are medical-ethical questions. Nor should we suppose that these questions are always the product of unusual circumstances. Medical-ethical questions arise from situations of everyday living, and the fact that we are not facing them now does not mean that we will not face them later. We meet them, for example, when dealing with an elderly relative suffering from acute senile dementia, or with a daughter in irreversible coma, or with an unborn child diagnosed as having a serious congenital defect. And in these situations we may well decide that the traditional imperative of prolonging life is no longer applicable. It is likely, however, that many will disagree with our decision.

3. THE PRINCIPLES OF MORAL ACTION: NORMATIVE ETHICS

Let us suppose, then, that there is no dispute about the facts of a particular case – that, for example, my grandmother is senile. Why, then, should there be a disagreement about what to do with her? The explanation, as we shall see, invariably lies in a disagreement between normative principles. When we attempt to provide standards or rules to help us distinguish right from wrong actions, or good from bad people, we are, as we saw earlier, engaged in normative ethics. In normative ethics, to repeat, we try to arrive by rational means at a set of acceptable criteria which will enable is to decide why any given action is 'right' or any particular person is called 'good.' But not surprisingly, the application of different principles leads to moral disagreement. Take, for example, the rule 'Thou shalt not kill.' Opponents of euthanasia appeal to this rule to support their claim that no one person, or group of people, has the right to take the life of another. Advocates of euthanasia, on the other hand, may refer to different standards: that, for example, such action may be justified if it reduces needless suffering. So behind the question, 'Should Mrs Smith be taken off the respirator?' lies a debate between rival theories of moral behaviour. Having justified the rule, we then apply it to the case at hand, namely to Mrs Smith. Again, the dispute here is not about Mrs Smith's medical condition, but about which normative rules should be applied to her case.

Normative ethics is generally split into two categories:

a) teleological theories
b) deontological theories

The philosopher C D Broad defined them in this way:

Deontological theories hold that there are ethical propositions of the form: 'Such and such a kind of action would always be right (or wrong) in such and such circumstances, no matter what its consequences might be.' Teleological theories hold that the rightness or wrongness of an action is always determined by its tendency to produce certain consequences which are intrinsically good or bad.[1]

1. **A teleological theory** (from the Greek *telos*, meaning 'end') maintains, therefore, that moral judgements are based entirely on the effects produced by an action. An action is considered right or wrong in relation to its *consequences*. This view appeals to our common sense. Often, when considering a course of action, we ask: 'Will this hurt me?' or 'Will this hurt others?' Thinking like this is thinking teleologically: whether we do something or not is determined by what we think the consequences will be, whether we think they will be good or bad. Inevitably, of course, people have different opinions about whether a particular result is good or bad, and this accounts for the great variety of teleological theories. For some, an action is only right if it benefits the person performing the action. For others, this is too narrow, and the action's effects must apply to others besides the agent.

2. **A deontological theory** denies what a teleological theory affirms. The rightness of an action does not depend solely on its consequences since there may be *certain features of the act itself* which determine whether it is right or wrong. Pacifists, for example, contend that the act of armed aggression is wrong and always will be wrong, no matter what the consequences. Others believe we should take account of the 'motive' behind the act. If the intention of the person performing the act was to do harm, then that action is wrong quite apart from its effects, harmful or not. Or again, many argue that certain actions are right if they conform to certain absolute rules, like 'Keep your promises' or 'Always tell the truth'. It is quite possible that, in obeying these rules, you do not promote the greatest possible balance of good over evil; but for the deontologist this does not detract from the original good of your action in keeping your promise or telling the truth.

1. *Five Types Of Ethical Theory*, London, Kegan Paul, Trench, Trubner & Co., 1930, pp.206-207.

As we shall see, this difference between the teleologist and the deontologist is the most fundamental one in normative ethics. Simply put, the former looks ahead to the consequences of his or her actions, while the latter looks back to the nature of the act itself. It is not, however, always easy to pigeonhole our everyday decisions in this way, and invariably we find that they are compounded of both teleological and deontological elements.

Exercise 2

Which of the following moral commands (which you may or may not agree with) are teleological, deontological, or both?

a. Do not drink and drive
b. Do not accept sweets from strangers
c. Do not take unnecessary risks
d. Always obey your superiors
e. Do not kill
f. Avenge wrongs done to you
g. Tell the truth
h. Never tell a lie except to an enemy
i. Love thy neighbour as thyself
j. Be ruled by your conscience
k. Never trust a traitor
l. Do not eat pork
m. Do not steal
n. Do not get caught stealing
o. Do as you would be done by

Exercise 3

Here are some examples of moral dilemmas. In each example: 1) justify your answer in relation to a particular moral principle; 2) determine whether this principle is teleological, deontological, or a mixture of both; 3) think of another situation, if you can, in which you would consider disobeying this principle.

1. A reluctant father

A father is asked to donate a kidney to his daughter, who is suffering from progressive renal failure. The father refuses on the grounds that he is afraid of the operation, that his daughter's prognosis is not good, and that she has suffered enough already. Because he does not want to be accused of causing his own daughter's death, the father asks the doctor to tell the family that his kidney is not compatible.
Should the doctor obey the father's request?

2. A Suspicious Nurse

A nurse suspects that a doctor is spending more time with some patients than others, and charging them privately for more sophisticated medication. A patient confirms to her that this has been happening. The nurse knows that if she tells the authorities the doctor will be dismissed for professional misconduct. On the other hand, he is a brilliant and popular man, who obtains remarkable results.

What should the nurse do?

3. A young boy

A young boy is totally comatose and unresponsive, although not brain dead. His parents argue that, even in this condition, his life is of supreme value to them, and they visit him every day. But they cannot pay for his expensive care, and the nurses feel that they would be better employed elsewhere. The boy contracts an infection which requires extensive antibiotic treatment. Should this treatment be given?

4. An old lady

After a car accident, an old lady in her late eighties is admitted to hospital. She is very independent-minded, and brought up her large family on her own. She makes it quite clear to the nurses that she wants to die, and so refuses to eat. Her children want to respect her wishes, but at the same time know that, if she eats and gains strength, she will soon be able to go home. Should she be force-fed?

5. A drug thief

Your colleague says: 'I have something important to tell you, but you must keep it a secret.' You promise you will. Your friend then confesses that it was he who stole the drugs from the surgery. 'But this is terrible,' you say. 'David has already been accused of this and has been sacked! You must own up at once!' Your friend refuses.

What should you do?

6. A surgeon

A surgeon is engaged in important research into the causes of kidney failure among infants. While removing the appendix of a small child, he also extracts a small piece of kidney, arguing that this is necessary if his research is to continue.

You are an assisting nurse. Should you report the surgeon?

7. An elderly person.

An elderly person is alone and incontinent, and, although her home is in a deplorable state, she refuses to leave. It is clear to her family that she must be admitted to a home.

Should her relatives deceive her by saying that she is 'going on a holiday'? Or should her resistance be overcome by tranquillizing drugs?

8. A young girl.
A young girl, aged fifteen, comes to you as her doctor. She wants you to supply her with contraceptives. You discuss the matter with her and discover that she has never had sexual intercourse before and has never discussed the matter with her family.
Should you prescribe the contraceptives or inform her parents?

Questions: Normative Ethics

1. How do ethical statements differ from ordinary empirical statements? Give examples.

2. List four qualities of human character that you think are good and four that are bad. Do you think them good and bad for deontological or teleological reasons?

3. Argue for a) pacifism and b) vegetarianism from both a deontological and teleological viewpoint.

4. Tom has lived alone on a desert island all his life. How would you explain to him the difference between right and wrong?

5. Are there any moral rules which you believe all societies, despite their cultural differences, should adopt? What are they, and how would you explain their universal acceptance?

Bibliography: Normative Ethics

Billington, Ray *Living Philosophy*, London & New York, Routledge, 1988. A wide-ranging discussion of normative theories, coupled with contemporary issues.

Brandt, R B *Ethical Theory: The Problem of Normative and Critical Ethics*, Englewood Cliffs, NJ: Prentice-Hall, 1959. Review of all major normative theories.

Broad, C D *Five Types of Ethical Theory*, London, Kegan Paul, Trench, Trubner & Co, 1930.

Frankena, William K *Ethics*, Englewood Cliffs, NJ: Prentice-Hall, 1973. A textbook, although not easy.

Gowans, Christopher W (ed.) *Moral Dilemmas*, Oxford, Oxford University Press, 1987. Standard anthology.

Grassian, Victor *Moral Reasoning*, Englewood Cliffs, NJ: Prentice-Hall, 1981. Combines analysis of normative theories with discussion of contemporary moral problems.

Hospers, John *Human Conduct*, New York: Harcourt Brace Jovanovich, 1972. An excellent introduction to major theories.

MacIntyre, Alasdair *A Short History of Ethics*, London, Routledge & Kegan
    Paul, 1968. A history from the Homeric age to present day.
Purtill, Richard *Thinking about Ethics*, Englewood Cliffs, NJ: Prentice-Hall,
    1976. A short but imaginative introduction.
Raphael, D D *Moral Philosophy*, Oxford, Oxford University Press, 1981. A
    short introduction.
Taylor, P W (ed.) *Problems of Moral Philosophy*, Belmont, Calif: Dickenson,
    1967. Substantial extracts, with introductions.

Medical Ethics

The following are useful introductory texts:

Beauchamp, Tom (with James Childress). *Principles of Biomedical Ethics*,
    4th ed., New York, Oxford University Press, 1994.
– (edited, with LeRoy Walters). *Contemporary Issues in Bioethics*, Encino,
    Calif., Dickenson Publishing Co., 1978.
Devettere, Raymond J. *Practical Decision Making in Health Care Ethics*,
    Washington, D.C., Georgetown University Press, 1995.
Mappes, Thomas (with Jane Zembatty). *Biomedical Ethics*, 3rd ed., New York,
    McGraw-Hill, 1991.
Munson, Robert. *Intervention and Reflection: Basic Issues in Medical Ethics*.
    4th ed., Belmont, Calif., Wadsworth Publishing Co., 1992)
Pence, Gregory E. *Classic Cases in Medical Ethics*, New York, McGraw-
    Hill, 1990
Sumner, L W (edited, with Joseph Boyle). *Philosophical Perspectives on
    Bioethics*, Toronto, University of Toronto Press, 1996.

Chapter 2
Egoism

WHAT IS EGOISM?

The first normative ethical theory I want to look at is *Egoism*. Of all ethical theories, egoism has received the worst press. This is because we tend to deplore the attitude of mind that egoists so often display – the attitude that says 'Look after Number One' or 'Do what you want to do.' Many people find this attitude devoid of moral worth, and close to what we commonly call 'selfishness.' Many thinkers and philosophers, however, have profoundly disagreed with this judgment. What we have here, they contend, is not something immoral but something quite natural and understandable; something, in fact, that contains a fundamental insight into the nature of human motivation – namely, that a human being, however much he or she may wish or seek to do otherwise, cannot do other than serve his or her own best interests.

Egoism, indeed, is one of the most popular and pervasive normative theories of moral behaviour. It maintains that *each person ought to act to maximise his or her own long-term good or well-being.* An egoist, in other words, is someone who holds that his one and only obligation is to himself and his only duty is to serve his own self-interest. Of course, different people have different ideas about what is or is not in their own interests. For a thief it might be to avoid capture, for a sailor to be able to swim. The fact, however, that people do have different ambitions is quite beside the point for egoists, and in no way affects the general theory they are propounding. They are not saying that everybody should have identical aims; all they are claiming is that each person should act if and only if that action serves to promote their own long-term interests. If an action produces benefits for them, they should do it; if it doesn't, then it is morally acceptable for them not to do it.

It follows from this that an egoist is not necessarily someone who is always seeking pleasure and excitement without a thought for the future. To suppose otherwise is to overlook the careful inclusion of the words 'long-term' in the previous definitions. Egoists are not necessarily short-sighted: they know very well that self-interest depends not only on immediate aims but also on long-term effects. After all, Smith may like to get drunk everyday, but this would hardly be serving his long-term interests, such as leading an active and healthy life. An egoist, then, is not what he or she appears to be at first: they do not believe that you should always do what you like when you like, for the simple reason that doing what you like may not, in the end, serve your own best interests.

Historically speaking, the clearest evidence that egoists are not straightforward pleasure-seekers is to be found in the career and teaching of the Greek philosopher Epicurus (341-270 BC). Epicurus was perhaps the most influential exponent of egoism in the late classical world, and from his name we derive the word 'epicure', i.e. a lover of good food and drink. Epicurus was also a **hedonist** (from the Greek *hedone*, meaning 'pleasure'): that is, he believed that pleasure alone was good and worth pursuing. From this, one might conclude that Epicurus was a man who dedicated himself to a life of pleasure, indulgence and excess. But the contrary was the case. He lived very simply and is said to have suffered from stomach trouble, requiring the blandest of food and drink ('Send me a cheese,' he wrote to a friend, 'that I may fare sumptuously'). In his teaching he was uncompromising. He condemned the pursuit of sensual desires and believed instead that long-term pleasure could best be achieved by philosophical and artistic contemplation, by a virtual absence of the physical appetites, and by a general freedom from worry or distress. Indeed, his own retiring style of life, simple and frugal as it was, suggests a total repudiation of the pursuit of pleasure at any cost. For Epicurus, the more violent a pleasure, the more likely were the unpleasant after-effects. So, in his *Letter to Menoeceus*, he writes:

> Pleasure is our first and kindred good. It is the starting-point of every choice and of every aversion, and to it we come back, inasmuch as we make feeling the rule by which to judge of every good thing. And since pleasure is our first and native good, for that reason we do not choose every pleasure whatsoever, but oft-times pass over many pleasures when a greater annoyance ensues from them. And oft-times we consider pains superior to pleasures when submission to the pains for a long time brings us as a consequence a greater pleasure. While, therefore, all pleasure, because it is naturally akin to us, is good, not all pleasure is choiceworthy, just as all pain is an evil and yet not all pain is against another, and by looking at the conveniences and inconveniences, that all these matters must be judged. Sometimes we treat the good as an evil, and the evil, on the contrary, as a good . . .
>
> When we say, then, that pleasure is the end and aim, we do not mean the pleasures of the prodigal or the pleasures of sensuality, as we are understood to do by some through ignorance, prejudice, or wilful misrepresentation. By pleasure we mean the absence of pain in the body and of trouble in the soul. It is not an unbroken succession of drinking-bouts and of revelry, not the sexual love, not the enjoyment of the fish and other delicacies of a luxurious table, which produces a pleasant life; it is sober reasoning, searching out the ground of every choice and avoidance, and banishing those beliefs through which the greatest good is prudence. Wherefore prudence is a more precious thing even than philosophy; from it spring all other virtues, for it teaches that we cannot lead a life of pleasure which is not also a life of prudence, honour, and justice; nor lead a life of prudence, honour, and justice, which is not also a life of pleasure. For the virtues have grown into one with a pleasant life, and a pleasant life is inseparable from them.[1]

In modern philosophical terms, Epicurus is here making a distinction between intrinsic good and instrumental good. Something is intrinsically good if it is worth having for its own sake; something is instrumentally good if, while not necessarily being good in itself, it leads to goodness. For Epicurus pleasure is the sole **intrinsic good** and everything else is a possible **instrumental good**.

1. Diogenes Laertius, The *Lives of the Eminent Philosophers*, trans. R D Hicks, Cambridge, Mass.: Harvard University Press, 1950, Vol. II, pp. 123-124.

This is not to say, however, that pleasure itself is always instrumentally good because there may be cases in which an immediate pleasure does not lead to a long-term pleasure. For example, alcohol brings an intrinsic good in that it brings pleasure, but it does not bring instrumental good because of its ultimate consequences. Amputation, on the other hand, brings no intrinsic good in itself but it may lead to it in bringing about the pleasures of recovery and health.

Exercise 1

How would you classify the following? Are they intrinsically good or bad or instrumentally good or bad? Give your reasons.

a.	Kindness	**i.**	Wealth
b.	Vaccination	**j.**	Envy
c.	Freedom	**k.**	Knowledge
d.	Beauty	**l.**	Loyalty
e.	Murder	**m.**	Obedience
f.	Doing one's duty	**n.**	Sadism
g.	Punishment	**o.**	Courage
h.	Revenge	**p.**	Disease
q.	Truth-telling	**r.**	Ambition

PSYCHOLOGICAL EGOISM

Many people are egoists because they believe egoism is the only ethical theory which presents an accurate account of what human beings are like. It rests, they claim, on a fundamental insight into the nature of man, or, to be more specific, on a psychological theory of human behaviour which is true. This theory is known as psychological egoism. It states that a *human being is psychologically incapable or doing anything that does not promote his or her own self-interest.*

Psychological egoism is not itself an ethical doctrine but a theory of human motivation: it is telling us how men are constructed, not whether their actions are right or wrong. For if psychological egoism is true, then any ethical system that suggests that we ought to do something which does not further our own self-interests will be false. Such a system is flying in the face of facts: it is asking people to do things they cannot do. The significance of psychological egoism is, therefore, that it requires the rejection of all ethical theories that are not themselves egoistic.

This connection between psychological egoism and ethics in general is best expressed in the saying 'Ought implies can'. If we say that somebody *ought* to perform a certain action, we are clearly implying that this person could do it if he wished: it is an action *possible* for him; he has a choice – to do it or not. But if this person simply cannot perform this action, no matter how hard he may try, then there is clearly no sense in our still saying that he ought to do it. After all, no one can be expected to do what they cannot do. If Smith cannot swim, he cannot save the drowning child. Should someone complain that Smith ought to have saved the child, Smith can reasonably reply that this accusation is absurd: he cannot be blamed for what he cannot do but only for not doing what he could do. Similarly, then, to say with psychological egoism that a person is psychologically able to perform only those actions which further his own self-interest implies that he cannot do otherwise, cannot be expected to do otherwise, and cannot be blamed if he does not do otherwise. So:

a. If what we ought to do is what we are capable of doing.
b. And if all we are capable of doing is furthering our own self-interest.
c. Then all that we ought to do is further our own self-interest.
d. Thus egoism is true.

We should be clear what is not being said here. Psychological egoism is not claiming that all people *behave* selfishly. The theory would not deny, for example, that some people devote their lives to helping others. What is being said, however, is that the motive behind such actions is always and ultimately selfish. In other words, while people often do benevolent acts (i.e. acts which help others), they cannot act benevolently (i.e. act for the sake of those being helped). Human beings are so constructed that they cannot help acting in their own interests even when they are helping others. Psychological egoism, therefore, does not exclude unselfish acts, only unselfish desires. This point is well-illustrated by the following story:

> Mr Lincoln once remarked to a fellow-passenger on an old-time mud coach that all men were prompted by selfishness in doing good. His fellow-passenger was antagonizing this position when they were passing over a corduroy bridge that spanned a slough. As they crossed this bridge they espied an old razor-backed sow on the bank making a terrible noise because her pigs had got into the slough and were in danger of drowning. As the old coach began to climb the hill, Mr Lincoln called out, 'Driver, can't you stop just a moment?' Then Mr Lincoln jumped out, ran back and lifted the little pigs out of the mud and water, and placed them on the bank. When he returned, his companion remarked: 'Now, Abe, where does selfishness come in on this little episode?' 'Why, bless your soul, Ed, that was the very essence of selfishness. I should have had no peace of mind all day had I gone on and left that suffering old sow worrying over those pigs. I did it to get peace of mind, don't you see?'[2]

Exercise 2

Consider whether the following situations are or are not examples of psychological egoism. Is it possible to regard them all as examples of it?

a. A man hurries to the scene of an accident, thinking 'One day it might be me!'

b. A doctor hurries to the scene of an accident, thinking 'Here is an opportunity to use my skill.'

2. Quoted by Victor Grassian, in *Moral Reasoning*, Englewood Cliffs, NJ.: Prentice-Hall, 1981, p.151.

c. A clergyman hurries to the scene of an accident, thinking 'God commands me to do this.'

d. A man sees a brick on the road and removes it, thinking 'There might have been an accident.' He does not drive himself and is leaving the country the next day.

e. The driver says to the policeman, who did not see the accident, 'It was my fault, officer!'

At one time psychological egoism was almost universally accepted by philosophers: now it is almost universally condemned. To understand why this is, let us look again at its central claim that 'All men serve their own self-interest.'

The first thing to remember about this claim is that it is not concerned with ethics but with human motivation: it is not commending certain courses of action so much as telling us what human beings are like and how they will inevitably act. A claim like this is called an empirical claim; that is, it gives information about the world, based on our experience of it ('empirical' comes from the Greek word for 'experience'). Thus an empirical proposition is considered true if it conforms to experience and observation, and false if it does not. The following are all empirical statements:

a. I have a nose
b. Norway has fjords
c. Some men have beards
d. All cats have whiskers

All these statements are considered true on the basis of available evidence. And the same evidence would make the following empirical statements false:

a. I have a beak
b. Norway has deserts
c. Some men have fins
d. All cats have wings

If, however, we look more closely at our four true statements, we see that they are not all equally verifiable according to the evidence. For while we would say of the first three propositions that they are conclusively verifiable – that is, there is sufficient evidence to demonstrate that they are true beyond rational doubt – we cannot say this of 'All cats have whiskers'. If we are to say that it is empirically true, then we must mean that it is true universally, that it is true of every single cat. But what observations could possibly verify such a claim? Clearly, none. However many cats we did observe, the possibility would always remain that we had not observed all cats. Some cats, indeed, we could not observe. What we have here, then, is an assumption about cats based on *what has so far been observed to be the case*. Thus, we must always allow for the possibility that around the corner lurks a whiskerless cat!

Once we realise that the central claim of psychological egoism is like the statement 'All cats have whiskers', we can see where its fatal weakness lies. The statement 'All men serve their own self-interest' is also an empirical generalization – a generalization about the nature of human conduct – and as such it is based on experience and observation. But how can this be? This claim is true only if there is evidence that there never has been and never could be any unselfish action; and this is evidence psychological egoists cannot provide. How can they be *certain* that the man who sacrifices his life for a friend is acting selfishly, or that the doctor running a leper colony does so through self-interest? Do they know these people that intimately? Is their knowledge of them sufficiently comprehensive? We cannot, of course, exclude the possibility that these people are selfishly motivated. But if the psychological egoist cannot provide evidence that they are, then he must allow for the possibility that they are not – and this possibility alone is sufficient to refute his proposition that all human beings serve their own self-interest.

Indeed, we may go further and say that this proposition, although claiming to be empirical, *is not an empirical proposition at all.* Empirical propositions are considered true or false on the basis of available evidence. The claim of psychological egoism, however, does not allow for its possible falsification. Let us take an example. Suppose X has to choose between two actions, A and B, where A is what we would ordinarily call a 'selfish' act and B an 'unselfish' act. If X chooses A, the psychological egoist will say that simply demonstrates the truth of his theory; but if X chooses B, the psychological egoist will not see this as contrary evidence and change his theory, but merely repeat that this choice must be selfish because X is a human being and all human beings act in this way. On this reasoning, therefore, it is not *evidence* which determines the theory but a *definition* of humankind, and a definition, moreover, that precludes any denial of its truth. To this extent, the claim that 'All human beings serve their own self-interest' is not empirical: it does not conform to the evidence but makes the evidence conform to it.

The criticisms offered here have done no more than point to the difficulties involved in general propositions of the sort 'All crows are black', 'All cats have whiskers' or 'All human beings serve their own self-interest', or indeed in any unqualified empirical proposition that includes words like 'any' or 'every'. If, as psychological egoists suppose, this quality of selfishness is inescapable, then men and women must be said to possess it *in all circumstances.* Psychological egoists are thus forced into the untenable position of having to affirm, first, that they have here completed a description of a particular object (human being) which foresees completely all the possible circumstances in which that description is true and in which it is false; and second, that their own factual knowledge of human beings is complete to the point that there is no chance of something unforeseen occurring (e.g. a person acting non-egoistically) that could upset or modify their description. This, however, is to assign to empirical knowledge an absoluteness it cannot possess.

ETHICAL EGOISM

While there are good reasons for supposing that psychological egoism is false, this does not mean that we should reject egoism out of hand. Indeed, there are many egoists who are equally critical of psychological egoism, who deny its claim to present an accurate analysis of man, and who are therefore quite ready to accept that people often do act against their own self-interest. Their point is, rather, that egoism, when properly understood, is not concerned with what motives men and women actually have but with those that they ought to have. In other words, the true strength of egoism lies in its ethical, not psychological, form and is thus best seen in that version of it known as **ethical egoism**. Ethical egoism maintains that *each person ought to act to serve his or her own self-interest.* This proposition, while agreeing that some people may act against their own interests, condemns such action when it occurs.

If ethical egoists do not depend on psychological egoism to justify their position, upon what do they depend? Undoubtedly part of their case is based on the belief that such a doctrine will produce a happier world. If greater happiness and reward come to those pursuing their own interest, then the more people do this the better. Such reasoning does not exclude actions ordinarily called 'moral' – for example, being honest, not stealing, helping your neighbour – but such actions are acceptable to the egoist only because they produce dividends for the agent, not because they are good or laudable in themselves: if you help others they will help you, if you don't steal neither will they; and so on.

Most of us are familiar with this type of argument and it is one often presented by both ancient and modern philosophers. Its classic form is found in the ethical teaching of Epicurus, to which we have already referred, and according to which the sole valid standard of right action is the avoidance of painful or unpleasant experiences. Its most famous proponent in modern philosophy is Thomas Hobbes (1588-1679). In his book *Leviathan* (1651) Hobbes writes that 'Good and evil are names that signify our appetites and aversions' – namely, that what we like or desire is good and what we dislike or wish to avoid is evil. This explains why the citizen places himself under an obligation to obey the law: it is not because the law is something good in itself but because it maintains the security of the individual by protecting him from the injury others might do him. Hence the obligation to obey the law is itself grounded on self-interest.

Exercise 3

You are the Managing Director of a pharmaceutical company. What are your decisions in the following cases and on what grounds would you make them?
Would you call these decisions egoistic? If not, why not?

Case 1. You discover that your product Y has unpleasant and even harmful side-effects, while your rival's product has none.
Do you stop production of Y?

Case 2. Your product Y is the only drug of its type available on the market, and many patients have benefited from it: some, however, have contracted cancer.

Do you stop production of Y?

Case 3. Your product Y is being tested for harmful side-effects. None have so far been found, but it cannot be sold at home until these tests are completed.

Meantime, do you market the drug abroad?

Case 4. You accept that your product Y is a potential cause of cancer. However, safety regulations in foreign countries are not so stringent.

Do you market the drug abroad?

Case 5. Your product Y, while safely used at home, is positively dangerous in underdeveloped countries, where often the standard of hygiene is low.

Do you market the drug in these countries?

Ethical egoism is not without its difficulties. A major criticism is that it contains an inner contradiction, it being contradictory to claim that *all* men and women should look after themselves if this results in my *not* looking after myself. For example, suppose both Jones and I have a particular disease and that we shall both die unless treated with a specific vaccine. Suppose further that there is only one phial of vaccine available. If I am an ethical egoist I must not only attempt to get the vaccine exclusively for myself but also recommend, should I be asked, that Jones do the same: I must recommend, in other words, that Jones serve his interests but not mine. But if I do this I contradict the basic principle of ethical egoism since I clearly would not be serving my best interests if I gave Jones this advice. It clearly cannot be to my advantage to convince him to serve his own interests when these interests destroy mine. Indeed, in this particular case, my best ploy would be to persuade him to forego his egoistic principles and adopt a more altruistic approach. Thus we arrive at the peculiar situation in which my interests as an ethical egoist are best served if I proclaim that ethical egoism is a *false doctrine*!

This line of attack on ethical egoism has been developed by the philosopher Kurt Baier. Ethical egoism, he says, cannot decide in cases where there is a *conflict of interests*. Consider the following case:

Let A and B be candidates for the presidency of a certain country and let it be granted that it is in the interest of either to be elected, but that only one can succeed. It would then be in the interest of B but against the interest of A if B were elected, and vice versa, and therefore in the interest of B but against the interest of A if A were liquidated, and vice versa. But from this it would follow that B ought to liquidate A, that it is wrong for B not to do so, that B has not 'done his duty' until he has liquidated A; and vice versa. Similarly A, knowing that his own liquidation is in the interest of B and therefore anticipating B's attempts to secure it, ought to take steps to foil B's endeavours. It would be wrong for him not to do so. He would 'not have done his duty' until he had made sure of stopping B. It follows that if A prevents B from liquidating him, his act must be said to be both wrong and not wrong – wrong because it is the prevention of what B ought to do, his duty, and wrong for B not to do it; not wrong because it is what A ought to do, his duty, and wrong for A not to do it. But one and the same act (logically) cannot be both morally wrong and not morally wrong. This is obviously absurd. For morality is designed to apply in just such cases, namely, those where interests conflict. But if the point of view of morality were that of self-interest, then there could never be moral solutions of conflicts of interest.[3]

The strength of Baier's criticism can be seen if we place ourselves in the position of a judge deciding a conflict of interest, in which A and B want the same thing (be it the presidency, the custody of a child, some land or whatever). If the judge is an ethical egoist, he will never be able to resolve the issue between A and B because both of them are, in his eyes, right to pursue their own interests and, moreover, right to pursue them by any means available, the means being justified by their self-interest. In this way the principle of ethical egoism not only makes it impossible to decide who has the rightful claim, but also legitimates any action – legal or illegal – which will be the method by which the person concerned attains their end.

As a further variation on this argument, it is worth noting that ethical egoists give advice irrespective of the particular worth or merit of the individual they are advising; that is, they make no moral judgment as to whether it would be *good* or *bad* if this individual did in fact achieve his aim – provided, of course, that this person's interest does not conflict with theirs. To take Baier's example: suppose you, as an ethical egoist, are advising A and B about obtaining the presidency, and suppose that it makes no personal difference to you who becomes president. Thus you advise A to liquidate B and B to liquidate A. When you are with A, his interests count; when with B, his interests count; but no judgement is here made as to whether it would be *better* if A and not B became president, and vice versa, for each man has an equal right to aim for the presidency, and this right is justified by the self-interest displayed. Thus you are deprived of the ability to decide who *ought* to be president. Hence there is an absence of moral decision. For as long as their interests do not disadvantage yours, you must remain neutral as to the rightness or wrongness of each man's candidacy, be he saint or sinner.

If the doctrine of self-interest cannot either judge or advise in cases of conflicting interest, then it is time to ask whether ethical egoism is an ethical system at all. Egoists, as we have seen, only have one principle – the promotion of their self-interest – so that what they *ought* to do is always what they think is best for them. Their understanding of what is right or wrong changes as their interest changes: at one moment a certain action will be applauded but at the next condemned. Such fluctuations in attitude render ethical egoism, as a theory of normative ethics, highly unsatisfactory. If an egoist thinks breaking the law is to his advantage, he will break it, even if this involves theft and murder; but this does not mean that he approves of crime but only that he

3. *The Moral Point of View*, Ithaca, NY: Cornell University Press, 1958, pp.189-190.

approves of it *in this instance*. No consistency of moral judgement can therefore be guaranteed. Finally, the reason why we invariably regard such actions as reprehensible, and thus find it hard to subscribe to any ethical system that permits them, is that they take no account of the happiness of those they affect. In a word, the theory of ethical egoism seems misguided because it ignores one apparently essential ingredient of morality: namely, that the normative principles of moral action are meant for everybody, equally and alike; that individuals have no privileges other than those which belong to the rest of mankind, and cannot accordingly set aside the interests of others in the pursuit of their own.

Exercise 4

One of the most famous arguments against morality is given in Plato's *Republic*. In this dialogue, Glaucon and Adeimanthus challenge Socrates to justify why a man should live a moral life. Their challenge is presented in the form of a story, known as the Myth of Gyges. Read the story and decide:

a) What you would do if you had Gyges' ring;
b) Give reasons for not using the ring.

The Myth of Gyges[4]

According to the tradition, Gyges was a shepherd in the service of the King of Lydia; there was a great storm, and an earthquake made an opening in the earth at the place where he was feeding his flock. Amazed at the sight, he descended into the opening, where, among other marvels, he beheld a hollow brazen horse, having doors, at which he, stooping and looking in, saw a dead body of stature, as appeared to him, more than human, and having nothing on but a gold ring; this he took from the finger of the dead and reascended. Now the shepherds met together, according to custom, that they might send their monthly report about the flocks to the king; into their assembly he came having the ring upon his finger, and as he was sitting among them he chanced to turn the collet of the ring inside his hand, when instantly he became invisible to the rest of the company and they began to speak of him as if he were no longer present. He was astonished at this, and again touching the ring he turned the collet outwards and reappeared; he made several trials of the ring, and always with the same result – when he turned the collet inwards he became invisible, when outwards he reappeared. Whereupon he contrived to be chosen one of the messengers who were sent to the court; where as soon as he arrived he seduced the queen, and with her help conspired against the king and slew him and took the kingdom. Suppose now that there were two such magic rings, and the just put on one of them and the unjust the other; no man can be imagined to be of such an iron nature that he would stand fast in justice. No man would keep his hands off what was not his own when he could safely take what he liked out of the market, or go into houses and lie with any one at his pleasure, or kill or release from prison whom he would, and in all respects be like a God among men. Then the actions of the just would be as the actions of the unjust; they would both come at last to the same point. And this we

---

4. Plato, *The Republic*, in *Five Great Dialogues*, trans. Benjamin Jowett, New York, Walter J. Black, 1942, pp.256-257.

may truly affirm to be a great proof that a man is just, not willingly or because he thinks that justice is any good to him individually, but of necessity, for wherever any one thinks that he can safely be unjust, there he is unjust. For all men believe in their hearts that injustice is far more profitable to the individual than justice, and he who argues as I have been supposing will say that they are right. If you could imagine any one obtaining this power of becoming invisible, and never doing any wrong or touching what was another's, he would be thought by the lookers-on to be a most wretched idiot, although they would praise him to one another's faces, and keep up appearances with one another from a fear that they too might suffer injustice.

Exercise 5

Another argument for egoism is presented by the contemporary philosopher Ayn Rand (1905-1982). In her novel *The Fountainhead*, the architect Howard Roark agrees to design a government housing project, Cortlandt Homes, for another architect, Peter Keating: his only requirement is that the project must be built exactly as he designed it. This agreement is broken and Roark dynamites the project. At his trial Roark defends his action. To what extent do you consider Roark's arguments legitimate?

Howard Roark's Speech[5]

The first right on earth is the right of the ego. Man's first duty is to himself. His moral law is never to place his prime goal within the persons of others. His moral obligation is to do what he wishes, provided his wish does not depend primarily upon other men. This includes the whole sphere of his creative faculty, his thinking, his work. But it does not include the sphere of the gangster, the altruist and the dictator.

A man thinks and works alone. A man cannot rob, exploit or rule – alone. Robbery, exploitation and ruling presuppose victims. They imply dependence. They are the province of the second-hander.

Rulers of men are not egoists. They create nothing. They exist entirely through the persons of others. Their goal is their subjects, in the activity of enslaving. They are as dependent as the beggar, the social worker and the bandit. The form of dependence does not matter.

But men were taught to regard second-handers – tyrants, emperors, dictators – as exponents of egoism. By this fraud they were made to destroy the ego, themselves and others. The purpose of the fraud was to destroy the creators. Or to harness them. Which is a synonym.

From the beginning of history, the two antagonists have stood face to face: the creator and the second-hander. When the first creator invented the wheel, the first second-hander responded. He invented altruism.

The creator – denied, opposed, persecuted, exploited – went on, moved forward and carried all humanity along on his energy. The second-hander contributed nothing to the process except the impediments. The context has another name: the individual against the collective . . .

Now, in our age, collectivism, the rule of the second-hander and second-rater, the ancient monster, has broken loose and is running amuck. It has brought men to

5. Ayn Rand, *The Fountainhead*, New York & Indianapolis, The Bobbs-Merril Co., 1943. This passage reprinted in Rand, *For the New Intellectual*, New York, Random House, 1961, pp.82-85.

a level of intellectual indecency never equalled on earth. It has reached a scale of horror without precedent. It has poisoned every mind. It has swallowed most of Europe. It is engulfing our country . . .

Now you know why I dynamited Cortlandt.

I designed Cortlandt. I gave it to you. I destroyed it.

I destroyed it because I did not choose to let it exist. It was a double monster. In form and in implication. I had to blast both. The form was mutilated by two second-handers who assumed the right to improve upon that which they had not made and could not equal. They were permitted to do it by the general implication that the altruistic purpose of the building superseded all rights and that I had no claim to stand against it.

I agreed to design Cortlandt for the purpose of seeing it erected as I designed it and for no other reason. That was the price I set for my work. I was not paid . .

I came here to say that I do not recognize anyone's right to one minute of my life. Nor to any part of my energy. Nor to any achievement of mine. No matter who makes the claim, how large their number or how great their need.

I wished to come here and say that I am a man who does not exist for others.

It had to be said. The world is perishing from an orgy of self-sacrificing. I wished to come here and say that the integrity of a man's creative work is of greater importance than any charitable endeavour. Those of you who do not understand this are the men who're destroying the world.

Questions: Egoism

1. What do you consider the three most important long-term pleasures?

2. What are the moral objections, if any, to the 'playboy'?

3. For Epicurus the avoidance of pain is more important than the acquisition of pleasure. In that case why not advocate (like the hedonist Hegesias) suicide on the grounds that it guarantees a state with no pain at all? Discuss.

4. Construct a moral situation to which you believe psychological egoism does not apply. Give your reasons.

5. Why is it claimed that the statement 'All men serve their own self-interest' is not an empirical statement?

6. Discuss and illustrate the conflict of interest within ethical egoism. Do you consider this conflict a decisive objection to the theory?

7. In what circumstances would you act immorally if you knew you could not be caught or punished?

8. 'To pursue one's own self-interest is good business practice: it creates jobs and raises the standard of living.' Discuss.

9. The company, of which you are Chairman, has discovered valuable mineral deposits. Would you purchase the land at the current market value, saying nothing to the present owner of its real worth?

10. Consider the following case. What other method of selection (if any) would you adopt? Would it make any difference if one crew-member had navigational experience?

The private yacht Mignonette sailed from Southampton on May 19, 1884, bound for Sydney, Australia, where it was to be delivered to its owner. There were four persons aboard, all members of the crew: Dudley, the captain; Stephens, mate; Brooke, seaman; and Parker, a 17 year-old cabin boy and apprentice seaman. The yacht went down in the South Atlantic and all put off in a 13 foot lifeboat. After twenty days in the boat, during which they had no fresh water except rain water and during the last eight of which they had no food, Dudley, with Stephen's assent, killed the boy. Brooke objected. Thereafter all three fed on the body of the boy for four days, On the fifth day they were rescued. According to the jury's verdict, there was no likelihood that any of them would have survived unless one were killed and eaten, and it so appeared to the men.[6]

Bibliography: Egoism

Baier, Kurt *The Moral Point of View*, Ithaca, NY: Cornell University Press, 1958. Chapter 8 contains an influential criticism of the theory.

Beauchamp, T L & Bowie, N E (eds)*Ethical Theory and Business*, Englewood Cliffs, NJ: Prentice-Hall, 1983) Important collection of essays on business ethics.

Gauthier, D P *The Logic of Leviathan*, Oxford, Clarendon Press, 1969. Chapter 2 discusses Hobbes' moral theory.

Grassian, Victor *Moral Reasoning*, Englewood Cliffs, NJ: Prentice-Hall, 1981. Chapter 7.

Laertius, Diogenes *The Lives of the Eminent Philosophers* trans. R D Hicks, Cambridge, Mass: Harvard University Press, 1950.

Norman, Richard *The Moral Philosophers*, Oxford, Clarendon Press, 1983. Especially Chapter 4.

Plato, *The Republic* in *Five Great Dialogues*, trans Benjamin Jowett, New York, Walter J Black, 1942.

Rand, Ayn *Atlas Shrugged*, New York, Random House, 1957.

– *For the New Intellectual,* New York, Random House, 1961.

– *The Fountainhead*, New York & Indianapolis, The Bobbs-Merril Co, 1943.

– *The Virtue of Selfishness*, New York, New American Library, 1964. Rand's most extended discussion of her theory.

Raiser, S J, Dyck A J & Curran, W J (eds) *Ethics in Medicine*, Cambridge, Mass: The MIT Press, 1977.

---

6. From *Ethics in Medicine*, ed. S J Reiser, A J Dyck and W J Curren, Cambridge, Mass. The MIT Press, 1997, p. 663.

Chapter 3
Discussion: Egoism and the Right to Life

THE RIGHT TO LIFE

It might be supposed that egoists, having once declared that everyone should further their long-term interests, go on to say that everyone has a **right to life**. For if one's principal duty is to serve oneself, then self-preservation must be a priority since without life there would be no self-interest to serve. This supposition, however, is false. Because egoism is a teleological theory of normative ethics, the egoist's attitude to his own right to life, and to that of other people, will depend on whether he believes this right brings him benefit. If it does not, this right should be withdrawn. Egoists may therefore require another's death to further their interests, or indeed their own death, if they believe that life is intolerable and brings them no advantage. So if I know that I am going to Auschwitz, I have the right to commit suicide. I even have the right to assist the suicide of someone else going there. Similarly, if I know that the death of an evil dictator will end the torture of innocent people, I have the right to assassinate him; and so on. In all these cases the morality of withdrawing any person's right to life, including my own, is being judged in terms of future benefit; and it is worth adding that governments tend to argue along similar lines. For the state does not regard the citizen's right to life as an absolute moral right but as a legal right, as something that can be withdrawn by legislation. Here one thinks of those cases in which individuals may be deprived of their lives for committing murder or in which their lives may be at risk in battle. Whether the state is justified in doing these things is, of course, another matter.

For the deontologist, on the other hand, the right to life is an inalienable right: it is something that cannot legitimately be taken away by another individual or group. Saying therefore that people have this right means that one is never morally justified in killing them and that the absolute wrongfulness of so doing is established independently of what may result. Thus a man may neither commit suicide, nor help another to kill himself, nor sacrifice himself for others, nor expect others to do the same for him, no matter how much he may desire it. This absolute right to life helps explain why so many of us think that killing people is wrong and always wrong, and why even those who do not think like this require very special reasons for approving it – for example war and self-defence. Both may well share the view that killing in itself is wrong, an evil, and contrary to the most basic instincts of man.

Not surprisingly, the question of whether man has or has not a right to life raises many serious moral problems. Two in particular deserve special attention. These are the problems of **abortion** and **euthanasia**.

THE RIGHT TO LIFE AND ABORTION

Many opponents of abortion argue as follows: All human beings have a right to life; the foetus is a human being; therefore the foetus has a right to life. Abortion, as a denial of this right, is accordingly morally wrong. Those who support abortion maintain, however, that the foetus is not a human being but a clump of cells, and that, even if it were a human being, its right to life may be outweighed by certain other rights possessed by the mother. These rights, as described by Judith Thomson in her celebrated essay, are the woman's right to self-defence and her right to control her own body. We shall return to these presently.

When exactly does human life begin? There have been many divergent opinions. In the past there was strong support for the ancient Stoic view that life begins at birth, an opinion largely supported by contemporary Judaism, but this view has become increasingly unpopular the more our knowledge of foetal development has increased and the more the distinction between the born and the unborn has been blurred by advances in foetal photography. Others have found greater significance in 'quickening', the moment when the mother feels her baby move; but this event, although doubtless of great emotional significance for the mother, is not regarded as significant for the growth of the foetus. A more common argument is to say that human life begins at conception. It is held that, since development from foetus to baby is continuous, it is purely arbitrary to choose any point other than conception as the moment when one becomes a person. But this conclusion does not follow. One could say the same thing about the development from acorn to oak, but this does not mean that acorns are oaks: a distinction can be made between them. Similarly, a fertilised egg is so unlike a person that, to suppose otherwise, is to stretch the meaning of 'person' beyond all normal usage. Hence the most accepted view, particularly among physicians, is to focus upon some interim point at which the foetus becomes 'viable', that is, potentially able to live outside the mother's womb, albeit with artificial aid. But this argument has its own weaknesses, the most glaring being that the date of viability changes: in English law it has been reduced from twenty-eight weeks to twenty-four, though some argued for eighteen weeks. Many find it offensive that whether one counts as a person depends on the shifting state of medical research.

In the first of the essays which follow, Judith Thomson accepts that the foetus is a person at conception. Anti-abortionists, as we have seen, claim that it follows from this that the foetus, like all human beings, has the right to life, and that no other right can outweigh this right. Thomson challenges this view by saying that there are in fact two rights which may override the right to life. The first is the woman's right of self-defence, in which the mother may end the life of the foetus if it threatens her own; and the second is the right of ownership to her own body, according to which she has the right to use her body in the way she wants and which may or may not include carrying a foetus to term. Unlike the right of self-defence, the right of ownership extends to cases where the mother's life is not in danger. For example, if the woman has taken no contraceptive precautions, she has assumed responsibility for the unborn foetus and ought not to withdraw support; but if she has taken all possible precautions, she cannot be held responsible and may thus legitimately deny the foetus the use of her body. To continue the pregnancy in these circumstances is an act of charity on her part, but not a duty, and one which she cannot reasonably be expected to perform if the disadvantages to herself are considerable.

The Roman Catholic philosopher, John Noonan, accepts that there are instances in which abortion is justified – he cites the cases of the cancerous uterus and the ectopic pregnancy – but argues that these instances do not justify the conclusion that, whenever the needs of the mother conflict with those of the foetus, we should always decide in favour of the mother. The right to an abortion cannot be construed, as Thomson seems to think, as a property-right, since one is not morally justified, in virtue of one's property rights, to expel a weak and helpless person from one's home if that brings about his certain death. That some abortions are necessary should therefore be taken as exceptions to this general rule. Do not deliberately injure your fellow human being. In these terms, once the humanity of the foetus is perceived, abortion is never right except in self-defence. Abortion, in other words, violates the principle of the equality of human lives.

For Laura Purdy and Michael Tooley the weakness of Noonan's position lies in his assumption that there are no morally relevant differences between the born and the unborn. This is not the case. For even though the foetus is biologically human, it is nonetheless not human in one important sense: it is not a 'person,' i.e. it is not something that is capable of desiring to continue existing as a subject of experiences and other mental states. Since, therefore, the right to life only devolves upon those who are persons, the foetus has no such right. Abortion cannot therefore infringe a right that the foetus does not possess, and accordingly abortion should be available on demand.

Extract 1: Judith Jarvis Thomson:
A Defense of Abortion[1]

I propose . . . that we grant that the foetus is a person from the moment of conception. How does the argument go from here? Something like this, I take it. Every person has a right to life. So the foetus has a right to life. No doubt the mother has a right to decide what shall happen in and to her body, everyone would grant that. But surely a person's right to life is stronger and more stringent than the mother's right to decide what happens in and to her body, and so outweighs it. So the foetus may not be killed; an abortion may not be performed.

It sounds plausible. But now let me ask you to imagine this. You wake up in the morning and find yourself back to back in bed with an unconscious violinist. A famous unconscious violinist. He has been found to have a fatal kidney ailment, and the Society of Music Lovers has canvassed all the available medical records and found that you alone have the right blood type to help. They have therefore

1. 'A Defense of Abortion' *Philosophy and Public Affairs*, I, No. 1 (Autumn 1971). Reprinted in *Moral Problems*, ed. James Rachels, New York & London, Harper & Row, 1979, pp. 130-150

kidnapped you, and last night the violinist's circulatory system was plugged into yours, so that your kidneys can be used to extract poisons from his blood as well as your own. The director of the hospital now tells you, 'Look, we're sorry the Society of Music Lovers did this to you – we would never have permitted it if we had known. But still, they did it, and the violinist now is plugged into you. To unplug you would be to kill him. But never mind, it's only for nine months. By then he will have recovered from his ailment, and can safely be unplugged from you.' Is it morally incumbent on you to accede to this situation? No doubt it would be very nice of you if you did, a great kindness. But do you have to? What if it were not nine months, but nine years? Or longer still? What if the director of the hospital says, 'Tough luck, I agree, but you've now got to stay in bed, with the violinist plugged into you, for the rest of your life. Because remember this. All persons have a right to life, and violinists are persons. Granted you have a right to decide what happens in and to your body, but a person's right to life outweighs your right to decide what happens in and to your body. So you cannot ever be unplugged from him.' I imagine you would regard this as outrageous, which suggests that something really is wrong with that plausible-sounding argument I mentioned a moment ago . . . .

Suppose you find yourself trapped in a tiny house with a growing child. I mean a very tiny house, and a rapidly growing child – you are already up against the wall of the house and in a few minutes you'll be crushed to death. The child on the other hand won't be crushed to death; if nothing is done to stop him from growing he'll be hurt, but in the end he'll simply burst open the house and walk out a free man. Now I could well understand it if a bystander were to say, 'There's nothing we can do for you. We cannot choose between your life and his, we cannot be the ones to decide who is to live, we cannot intervene.' But it cannot be concluded that you too can do nothing, that you cannot attack it to save your life. However innocent the child may be, you do not have to wait passively while it crushes you to death. Perhaps a pregnant woman is vaguely felt to have the status of a house, to which we don't allow the right of self-defense. But if the woman houses the child, it should be remembered that she is a person who houses it.

I should perhaps stop to say explicitly that I am not claiming that people have a right to do anything whatever to save their lives. I think, rather, that there are drastic limits to the right of self-defense. If someone threatens you with death unless you torture someone else to death, I think you have not the right, even to save your life, to do so. But the case under consideration here is very different. In our case there are only two people involved, one whose life is threatened, and one who threatens it. Both are innocent: the one who is threatened is not threatened because of any fault, the one who threatens does not threaten because of any fault. For this reason we may feel that we bystanders cannot intervene. But the person threatened can . . . .

Where the mother's life is not at stake, the argument I mentioned at the outset seems to have a much stronger pull. 'Everyone has a right to life, so the unborn person has a right to life.' And isn't the child's right to life weightier than anything other than the mother's own right to life, which she might put forward as ground for an abortion. This argument treats the right to life as if it were unproblematic. It is not, and this seems to be precisely the source of the mistake.

For we should now ask what it comes to, to have a right to life. In some views, having a right to life includes having a right to be given at least the bare minimum one needs for continued life. But suppose that what in fact is the bare minimum a man needs for continued life is something he has no right at all to be given? . . . To return to the story I told earlier, the fact that for continued life that violinist needs the continued use of your kidneys does not establish that he has a right to be given the continued use of your kidneys. He certainly has no right against you that you should give him continued use of your kidneys. For nobody has any right to use your kidneys unless you give him such a right; and nobody has the right against you that you shall give him this right. If you do allow him to go on using your kidneys, this a kindness on your part, and not something he can claim from you as his due. Nor has he any right against the Society of Music Lovers that they should plug him into you in the first place. And if you now start to unplug yourself, having learned that you will otherwise have to spend nine years in bed with him, there is nobody in the world who must try to prevent you, in order to see to it that he is given something he has a right to be given. . . .

There is another way to bring out the difficulty. In the most ordinary sort of case, to deprive someone of what he has a right to is to treat him unjustly. Suppose a boy and his small brother are jointly given a box of chocolates for Christmas. If the older boy takes the box and refuses to give his brother any of the chocolates, he is unjust to him, for the brother has been given a right to half of them. But suppose that, having learned that otherwise it means nine years in bed with that violinist, you unplug yourself from him. You surely are not being unjust to him, for you gave him no right to use your kidneys, and no one else can have given him any such right. But we have to notice that in unplugging yourself, you are killing him; and violinists, like everybody else, have a right to life, and thus, in the view we were considering just now, the right not to be killed. So here you do what he supposedly has a right you shall not do, but you do not act unjustly to him in doing it.

The emendation which may be made at this point is this: the right to life consists not in the right not to be killed, but rather in the right not to be killed unjustly . . . . But if this emendation is accepted, the gap in the argument against abortion stares us plainly in the face: it is by no means enough to show that the foetus is a person, and to remind us that all persons have a right to life – we need to be shown also that killing the foetus violates its right to life, i.e. that abortion is unjust killing. And is it?

I suppose we may take it as a datum that in a case of pregnancy due to rape the mother has not given the unborn person a right to the use of her body for food and shelter. Indeed, in what pregnancy could it be supposed that the mother has given the unborn person such a right? It is not as if there were unborn persons drifting about the world, to whom a woman who wants a child says 'I invite you in.'

But it might be argued that there are other ways one can have acquired a right to the use of another person's body than by having been invited to use it by that person. Suppose a woman voluntarily indulges in intercourse, knowing of the chance it will issue in pregnancy, and then she does become pregnant; is she not in part responsible for the presence, in fact the very existence, of the unborn person inside? No doubt she did not invite it in. But doesn't her partial responsibility for its being there itself give it a right to the use of her body? If so, then her aborting it would be more like the boy's taking away the chocolates, and less like your unplugging yourself from the violinist – doing so would be depriving it of what it does have a right to, and thus would be doing it an injustice.

And then, too, it might be asked whether or not she can kill it even to save her own life: If she voluntarily called it into existence, how can she now kill it, even in self-defense?

The first thing to be said about this is that it is something new. Opponents of abortion have been so concerned to make out the independence of the foetus, to establish that it has a right to life, just as its mother does, that they have tended to overlook the possible support they might gain from making out that the foetus is dependent on the mother; in order to establish that she has a special kind of responsibility for it, a responsibility that gives it rights against her which are not possessed by any independent person.

On the other hand, this argument would give the unborn person a right to its mother's body only if her pregnancy resulted from a voluntary act, undertaken in full knowledge of the chance a pregnancy might result. It would leave out entirely the unborn person whose existence is due to rape. Pending the availability of some further argument, then, we would be left with the conclusion that unborn persons whose existence is due to rape have no right to the use of their mothers' bodies; so aborting them is not depriving them of anything they have a right to and hence is not unjust killing.

We should also notice that it is not at all plain that this argument really does go even as far as it seems to. For there are cases and cases, and the details make a difference. If the room is stuffy, and I therefore open a window to air it, and a burglar climbs in, it would be absurd to say, 'Ah, now he can stay, she's given him a right to the use of her house – for she is partially responsible for his presence there, having voluntarily done what enabled him to get in, in full knowledge that there are such things as burglars, and that burglars burgle.' It would be even more absurd to say this if I had had bars installed outside my windows, precisely to prevent burglars from getting in, and a burglar got in only because of a defect in the bars. It remains equally absurd if we imagine it is not a burglar who climbs in, but an innocent person who blunders or falls in. Again, suppose it were like this: people-seeds drift about in the air like pollen, and if you open your windows, one may drift in and take root in your carpets and upholstery. You don't want children, so you fix up your windows with fine mesh screens, the very best you can buy. As can happen, however, and on very, very rare occasions does happen, one of the screens is defective; and a seed drifts in and takes root. . . . Someone may argue that you are responsible for its rooting, that it does have a right to your house, because after all you could have lived out your life with bare floors and furniture, or with sealed windows and doors. But this won't do – for by the same token, anyone can avoid a pregnancy due to rape by having a hysterectomy.

There is room for yet another argument: We must surely all grant that there may be cases in which it would be morally indecent to detach a person from your body at the cost of his life. Suppose you learn that what the violinist needs is not nine years of your life, but only one hour. . . . Admittedly you were kidnapped. Admittedly you did not give anyone permission to plug him into you. Nevertheless, it seems to me plain that you ought to allow him to use your kidneys for that one hour – it would be indecent to refuse. . . . Now some people are inclined to use the term 'right' in such a way that it follows from the fact that you ought to allow a person to use your body for the hour he needs, that he has a right to use your body for the hour he needs, even though he has not been given that right by any person or act. . . . Suppose that box of chocolates I mentioned earlier had not been given to both boys jointly, but was given only to the older boy. There he sits, stolidly eating his way through the box, his small brother watching enviously. Here we are likely to say 'You ought not to be so mean. You ought to give your brother some of those chocolates.' My own view is that it just does not follow from the truth of this that the little brother has any right to any of the chocolates. If the boy refuses to give his brother any, he is greedy, stingy, callous – but not unjust. I suppose that the people I have in mind will say it does follow that the brother has a right to some of the chocolates, and thus that the boy does act unjustly if he refuses to give his brother any. But the effect of saying this is to obscure what we should keep distinct, namely the difference between the boy's refusal in this case and the boy's refusal in the earlier case, in which the box was given to both boys jointly, and in which the small brother thus had what was from any point of view clear title to half . . .

So my own view is that even though you ought to let the violinist use your kidneys for the one hour he needs, we should not conclude that he has a right to do so. We should say that if you refuse, you are, like the boy who owns all the chocolates and will give none away, self-centered and callous, indecent in fact, but not unjust. Similarly, that even supposing a case in which a woman pregnant due to rape ought to allow the unborn person to use her body for the hour he needs, we should not conclude that he has a right to do so; we should conclude that she is self-centered, callous, indecent, but not unjust, if she refuses. The complaints are no less grave; they are just different. However, there is no need to insist on this point. If anyone does wish to deduce 'he has a right' from 'you ought', then he must surely grant that there are cases in which it is not morally required of you that you allow that violinist to use your kidneys, and in which he does not have a right to use them, and in which you do not do him an injustice if you refuse.

And so also for mother and unborn child. Except in such cases as the unborn person has a right to demand it – and we were leaving open the possibility that there may be such cases – nobody is morally required to make large sacrifices, of health, of all other interests and concerns, of all other duties and commitments, for nine years, or even nine months, in order to keep another person alive.

Extract 2: John T Noonan: How to Argue about Abortion[2]

(Thomson's) ingenious attempt to make up a parallel to pregnancy imagines a kidnapping; a serious operation performed on the victim of the kidnapping; and a continuing interference with many of the activities of the victim. It supposes that violinist and victim were unrelated. It supposes nothing by which the victim's initial aversion to his yoke-mate might be mitigated or compensated. It supposes no degree of voluntariness. The similitude to pregnancy is grotesque. It is difficult to think of another age or society in which a caricature of this sort could be seriously put forward as a paradigm illustrating the moral choice to be made by a mother.

While Thomson focuses on this fantasy, she ignores a real case from which American tort law has generalized. On a January night in Minnesota, a cattle buyer, Orlando Depue, asked a family of farmers, the Flateaus, with whom he had dined, if he could remain overnight at their house. The Flateaus refused and, although Depue was sick and had fainted, put him out of the house into the cold night. Imposing liability of the Flateaus for Depue's loss of his frost-bitten fingers the court said, 'In the case at bar defendants were under no contract obligation to minister to plaintiff in his distress; but humanity demanded they do so, if they understood and appreciated his condition. . . . The law as well as humanity required that he not be exposed in his helpless condition to the merciless elements.'[3] Depue was a guest for supper although not a guest after supper. The American Law Institute, generalizing, has said that it makes no difference whether the helpless person is a guest or a trespasser. He has the privilege of staying. His host has the duty not to injure him or put him into an environment where he becomes nonviable. The obligation arises when one person 'understands and appreciates' the condition of the other.[4] Although the analogy is not exact, the case seems

---

2. Published by the Ad Hoc Committee in Defense of Life, reprinted in *Contemporary Issues in Bioethics*, edited with Introductions by T L Beauchamp and LeRoy Walters, Dickenson Publishing Co., Encino, CA, 1978, pp. 210-217

3. Depue v. Flateau, 100 Minn. 299, 111 W. W. 1(1907).

4. American Law Institute, *Restatement of Torts, Second* (1965) sec. 197

closer to the mother's situation than the case imagined by Thomson; and the emotional response of the Minnesota judges seems to be a truer reflection of what humanity requires. . . .

In the presentation of permissive abortion to the American public, major emphasis has been put on situations of great pathos – the child deformed by thalidomide, the child affected by rubella, the child known to suffer from Tay-Sachs disease or Downs syndrome, the raped adolescent, the exhausted mother of small children. These situations are not imagined, and the cases described are not analogies to those where abortion might be sought; they are themselves cases to which abortion is a solution. Who could deny the poignancy of their appeal?

Hard cases make bad law, runs the venerable legal adage, but it seems to be worse law if the distress experienced in situations such as these is not taken into account. If persons are to be given pre-eminence over abstract principle, should not exceptions for these cases be made in the most rigid rule against abortion? Does not the human experience of such exceptions point to a more sweeping conclusion – the necessity of abandoning any uniform prohibition of abortion, so that all the elements of a particular situation may be weighted by the woman in question and her doctor?

So far, fault can scarcely be found with this method of argumentation, this appeal to common experience. But the cases are over-simplified if focus is directed solely on the parents of a physically defective child or on the mother in the cases of rape or psychic exhaustion. The situations are very hard for the parents or the mother; they are still harder for the fetus who is threatened with death. If the fetus is a person as opponents of abortion contend, its destruction is not the sparing of suffering by the sacrifice of a principle but by the sacrifice of a life. Emotion is a proper element in moral response, but to the extent that the emotion generated by these cases obscures the claims of the fetus, this kind of argumentation fosters erroneous judgment.

In three of the cases – the child deformed by drugs, disease, or genetic defect – the neglect of the child's point of view seems stained by hypocrisy. Abortion is here justified as putting the child out of the misery of living a less than normal life. The child is not consulted as to the choice. Experience, which teaches that even the most seriously incapacitated prefer living to dying, is ignored. The feelings of the parents are the actual consideration, and these feelings are treated with greater tenderness that the fetal desire to live. The common unwillingness to say frankly that the abortion is sought for the parents' benefit is testimony, unwillingly given, to the intuition that such self-preference by the parents is difficult for society or for the parents themselves to accept.

The other kind of hard case does not mask preference for the parent by a pretence of concern for the fetus. The simplest situation is that of a pregnancy due to rape – in presentations to some legislatures it was usual to add a racist fillip by supposing a white woman and a black rapist – but this gratuitous pandering to bias is not essential. The fetus, unwanted in the most unequivocal way, is analogized to an invader of the mother's body – is it even appropriate to call her a mother when she did nothing to assume the special fiduciary cares of motherhood? If she is prevented from having an abortion, she is being compelled for nine months to be reminded of a traumatic assault. Do not her feelings override the right to life of her unwanted tenant?

Rape arouses fear and a desire for revenge, and reference to rape evokes emotion. The emotion has been enough for the state to take the life of a rapist.[5] Horror of the crime is easily extended to horror of the product, so that the fetal life becomes forfeit too. If horror is overcome, adoption appears to be a more humane

---

5. See Note, 'Constitutional Law: Capital Punishment for Rape Constitutes Cruel and Unusual Punishment When No Life is Taken or Endangered,' *Minnesota Law Review*, 1995 (1971) p.56.

solution than abortion. If the rape case is not being used as a stalking horse by proponents of abortion – if there is a desire to deal with it in itself – the solution is to assure the destruction of the sperm in the one to three days elapsing between insemination and impregnation.

Generally, however, the rape case is presented as a way of suggesting a general principle, a principle which could be formulated as follows: Every unintended pregnancy may be interrupted if its continuation will cause emotional distress to the mother. Pregnancies due to bad planning or bad luck are analogized to pregnancies due to rape; they are all involuntary [6]. Indeed many pregnancies can without great difficulty be assimilated to the hard case, for how often do persons undertake an act of sexual intercourse consciously intending that a child be the fruit of that act? Many pregnancies are unspecified by a particular intent, are unplanned, are in this sense involuntary. Many pregnancies become open to termination if only the baby consciously sought has immunity.

This result is unacceptable to those who believe that the fetus is human. It is acceptable to those who do not believe the fetus is human, but to reach it they do not need the argument based on the hard case. The result would follow immediately from the mother's dominion over a portion of her body. Opponents of abortion who out of consideration for the emotional distress caused by rape will grant the rape exception must see that the exception can be generalized to destroy the rule. If, on the other grounds they believe the rule good, they must deny the exception which eats it up. . . .

Defenders of an absolute prohibition of abortion have excepted the removal of a fertilized ovum in an ectopic pregnancy and the removal of a cancerous uterus containing an embryo. They have characterized the abortion as 'indirect.' They have meant that the surgeon's attention is focused on correcting a pathological condition dangerous to the mother and he only performs the operation because there is no alternative way of correcting it.[7] But the physician has to intend to achieve not only the improvement of the mother but the performance of action by which the fertilized ovum becomes nonviable. He necessarily intends to perform an abortion, he necessarily intends to kill. To say that he acts indirectly is to conceal what is being done. It is a confusing and improper use of the metaphor.[8]

A clearer presentation of the cases of the cancerous uterus and the ectopic pregnancy would acknowledge them to be true exceptions to the absolute inviolability of the fetus. Why are they not exceptions which would eat up the rule? It depends on what the rule is considered to be. The principle that can be discerned in them is, whenever the embryo is a danger to the life of the mother, an abortion is permissible. At the level of reason nothing more can be asked of the mother. The exceptions do eat up any rule preferring the fetus to the mother – any rule of fetus first. They do not destroy the rule that the life of the fetus has precedence over other interests of the mother. The exceptions of the ectopic pregnancy and the cancerous uterus are special cases of the general exception to the rule against killing, which permits one to kill in self-defence. Characterization of this kind of killing as 'indirect' does not aid analysis.

It is a basic intuition that one is not responsible for all the consequences of one's acts. By living at all one excludes others from the air one breathes, the food one eats. One cannot foresee all the results which will flow from any given action. It is imperative for moral discourse to be able to distinguish between injury foreseeably inflicted on another, and the harm which one may unknowingly bring about. . . .

6. See above, Thomson, p.35

7. See my 'An Almost Absolute Value in History,' Noonan, ed., *The Morality of Abortion*, Cambridge, Mass., Harvard University Press, 1970, pp.46-50.

8. To say that the act is in itself good seems to me to be an impossible supposition – there is no human act 'in itself' apart from intent. See for a contrary analysis, Germian Grisez, *Abortion: The Myths, The Realities, and the Arguments*, Washington, Corpus Books, 1970, p.329

In making moral judgments we respond to those human beings whom we see. . . . Look at the fetus, say the anti-abortionist, and you will see humanity. How long, they ask, can a man turn his head and pretend that he just doesn't see? . . . Is there a contradiction in the opponents of abortion appealing to perception when fetuses are normally invisible? Should one not hold that until beings are seen they have not entered the ranks of society? Falling below the threshold of sight, do not fetuses fall below the threshold of humanity? If the central moral transaction is response to the other person, are not fetuses peculiarly weak subjects to elicit our response? These questions pinpoint the principal task of the defenders of the fetus to make the fetus visible. Their task is different only in degree from that assumed by defenders of other persons who have been or are 'overlooked.' For centuries, color acted as a psychological block to perception, and the blindness induced by color provided a study basis for discrimination. Minorities of various kinds exist today who are 'invisible' and therefore unlikely to be 'heard' in the democratic process. Persons literally out of sight of society in prisons and mental institutions are often not 'recognized' as fellow humans by the world with which they have 'lost touch.' In each of these instances those who seek to vindicate the rights of the unseen must begin by calling attention to their existence. 'Look' is the exhortation they address to the callous and the negligent.

Perception of fetuses is possible with not substantially greater effort than that required to pierce the physical or psychological barriers to recognizing other human beings. The main difficulty is everyone's reluctance to accept the extra burdens of care imposed by an expansion of the numbers in whom humanity is recognized. It is generally more convenient to have to consider one's kin, one's peers, one's country, one's race. Seeing requires personal attention and personal response. The emotion generated by identification with a human form is necessary to overcome the inertia which is protected by a vision restricted to a convenient group. If one is willing to undertake the risk that more will be required in one's action, fetuses may be seen in multiple ways circumstantially, by the observation of a pregnant woman; photographically, by pictures of life in the womb; scientifically, in accounts written by investigators of prenatal life and child psychologists; visually, by observing a blood transfusion or an abortion while the fetus is alive or by examination of a fetal corpse after death. The proponent of abortion is invited to consider the organism kicking the mother, swimming peacefully in amniotic fluid, responding to the prick of an instrument, being extracted from the womb, sleeping in death. Is the kicker or swimmer similar to him or to her? Is the response to pain like his or hers? Will his or her own face look much different in death?. . .

Vicarious experience appears strained to the outer limit when one is asked to consider the experience of the fetus. No one remembers being born, no one knows what it is like to die. Empathy may, however, supply for memory, as it does in other instances when we refer to the experience of infants who cannot speak or to the experience of death by those who cannot speak again. The experience of the fetus is no more beyond our knowledge than the experience of the baby and the experience of dying.

Extract 3: Laura Purdy and Michael Tooley: Is Abortion Murder?[9]

This essay deals with the morality of abortion. We shall argue that abortion is morally unobjectionable, and that society benefits if abortion is available on demand. We begin by setting out a preliminary case in support of the practice of

9. *Abortion: Pro and Con*, edited by Robert L Perkins, Cambridge, Mass., Schenkman, 1974, pp. 129-136, 144-148.

abortion. . . . We conclude by considering what properties something needs in order to have a serious right to life, and we show that a human fetus does not possess those properties. Thus since there is no moral objection to abortion, the practice must be viewed as both permissible and desirable. . . .

Most anti-abortionist's feel that there are moral considerations involved in the issue of abortion that far outweigh considerations of human happiness. In view of what is at stake, this is not a claim to be lightly advanced. By lobbying for the prohibition of abortion, the anti-abortionist is in effect assuming responsibility for the consequences of those actions... (These) consequences are deeply disturbing. If anti-abortionists prohibit abortion, they will be responsible for untold human misery. They will be responsible for lessened enjoyment of sex; for frustration caused by inconvenient pregnancies and childbearing; for ill health, either physical or mental, of mothers or other persons; for deaths of women resulting from pregnancies and illegal abortions; for child abuse; for crimes committed by frustrated or improperly socialized individuals; and for the stunted life of everyone if overpopulation seriously curbs our freedom or lowers the quality of life. The ardent anti-abortionist must shoulder the burden of responsibility for these things since, had he acted otherwise, they would not have existed. What considerations, then, can the anti-abortionist point to that outweigh the suffering produced by the prohibition of abortion?

In reply to the accusation that the responsibility for this catalogue of woes lies on his shoulders, the anti-abortionist will argue that these evils are necessary in order to avoid a much greater evil. Fetuses have a right to life. They have a right to be born and to have the opportunity to become adults. To destroy them by abortion is seriously wrong, and in comparison with it the miseries enumerated above pale into insignificance. Fetuses are human beings, and to kill a human being is murder. . . .

Our view is as follows: an organism can have a right to life only if it now possesses, or possessed at some time in the past, the capacity to have a desire for continued existence. An organism cannot satisfy this requirement unless it is a person, that is, a continuing subject of experience and other mental states, and unless it has the capacity for self-consciousness – where an organism is self-conscious only if it recognizes that it is itself a person.

The basis for our contention is the claim that there is a conceptual connection between, on the one hand, the rights an individual can have and the circumstances under which they can be violated, and, on the other, the desires he can have. A right is something that can be violated and, in general, to violate an individual's right to something is to frustrate the corresponding desire. Suppose, for example, that someone owns a car. Then you are under a *prima facie* obligation not to take it from him. However, the obligation is not unconditional: if he does not care whether you drive off with his car, then *prima facie* you do not violate his right by doing so.

A precise formulation of the conceptual connection in question would require considerable care. The most important point is that violation of an individual's right to something does not always involve thwarting a *present* desire, that is, a desire that exists at the same time as the action that violates the right. Sometimes the violation of a right involves thwarting a *past* desire. The most dramatic illustration is provided by the rights of dead persons, since here the individual whose right is being transgressed no longer exists. When a person is unconscious, he does not have any desires. Yet his rights can certainly be infringed upon. This presents no problem when one takes past desires into account. The reason that it is wrong to kill a temporarily unconscious adult is that in the period before he became unconscious, he had a desire to go on living – a desire which it is possible to satisfy.

Violation of an individual's right may also involve frustrating a *future* desire. The most vivid example of this is the case of rights of future generations. Most people would hold that for those living today to use up all of the world's resources would violate the rights of future individuals. Here, as in the case of the rights of a dead person, the violation of an individual's rights occurs at a time when the individual does not even exist.

However, it is very important to notice that what is relevant are the desires that individuals will *actually have* at some time in the future. The desires that individuals would have *if* they were to exist at certain times at which, as a matter of fact, they will not exist, are not relevant. . . . Rights of future generations provide . . . an example. Suppose we know with certainty that no future generation will ever exist. Then there is no objection to using up the world's resources now. But if one were obliged to take into account the desires future individuals would have if they were to exist, it would be wrong to use up the world's resources.

A complete account of the connection between rights and desires would also have to take into consideration unusual cases, where an individual is in an emotionally unbalanced state, or where a person's desires have been affected by lack of relevant information, or by his being subjected to abnormal physiological or psychological factors. We shall ignore these, and confine ourselves to paradigm cases of violations of an individual's rights. When this is done, we can say that first, an individual cannot have a right to something unless there can be actions that would violate it. Second, an action cannot violate an individual's right to something unless it wrongs him by depriving him of the thing in question. And thirdly, an action can wrong an individual by depriving him of something only if it violates his desire for that thing. The desire is generally a present desire, but it may be a past or future desire. It follows that a person cannot have a right to something unless he is at some time capable of having the corresponding desire.

Let us now apply this to the case of the right to life. The expression 'right to life' misleads one into thinking that the right concerns the continued existence of a biological organism. The following example shows that this interpretation is inadequate. Suppose that we could completely reprogram an adult human so that it has (apparent) memories, beliefs, desires, and personality traits radically different from those associated with it before the reprogramming. (Billy Graham is reprogrammed as a replica of Bertrand Russell.) In such a case, however beneficial the change might be, it is true that *someone* has been destroyed, that someone's right to life has been violated, even though no biological organism has been killed. So the right to life cannot be construed as merely the right of a biological organism to continue to exist.

How then can the right in question be more accurately described? A natural suggestion is that the expression 'right to life' refers to the right of a person – a subject of experiences and other mental states – to continue to exist. However, this interpretation begs the question against certain possible positions. It might be that while persons have a right to continue to exist, so do other things that are only potentially persons. A right to life on this view would be either the right of a person to continue to exist or the right of something that is only potentially a person to become a person.

We concluded above that something cannot have a specific right unless it is capable at some time of having the corresponding desire. It follows from this together with the more accurate analysis of the right to life that something cannot have a right to life unless it is capable at some time either of having a desire to continue to exist as a person, or of having a desire to become a person. If something has not been capable of having either of these desires in the past, and is not now capable, then if it is now destroyed, it will never have possessed the capacity in question. Hence an organism cannot have a right to life unless it is now capable, or was capable at some time in the past, of having a desire to continue to exist as a person or a desire to become a person.

But recall now the discussion of desires (above). We showed that one's desires are limited by the concepts one possesses. Therefore one cannot have a desire to continue to exist as a person or a desire to become a person unless one has the concept of a person. The question we must now ask is whether something that is not itself a person could have the concept of such an entity. It seems plausible to hold that it could not. This means that something that is not a person cannot have a desire to become a person. Hence the right to life is confined to persons.

This brings us to our final requirement: an organism cannot have a right to life unless it is capable of self-consciousness, where an organism is self-conscious only if it recognizes that it is itself a continuing subject of experiences and other mental states. To justify this requirement, let us ask whether a person can fail to recognize that it is a person. If the answer were negative, it would follow from the requirement just established that an organism cannot have a right to life unless it possesses self-consciousness.

It is unclear, however, that something necessarily possesses self-consciousness if it is a person. Perhaps a person might fail to notice this fact about himself. Even if this is possible, it seems reasonable to believe that if something is a person, then it is *ipso facto capable* of acquiring the concept of a person, and of recognizing that it is itself a person. Thus even if something can have a right to life without having been self-conscious, it appears that it cannot have such a right without ever having possessed the capacity for self-consciousness.

Thus, the psychological characteristics that bestow a right to life upon an organism are these: it must be a person, capable of self-consciousness, of envisaging a future for itself, and of having desires about its own future states. . . .

The issue of abortion thus ceases to be puzzling. A human fetus does not have a right to life because it does not have the capacity for self-consciousness: it cannot conceive of itself as a continuing subject of experiences; it cannot envisage a future for itself, nor have the desires about such a future. A fetus is not a person, but only a potential person. Hence there is no moral objection to abortion. To prohibit it is to inflict unjustified suffering and death upon society.

Questions: Abortion

1. Consider this argument against Thomson: While the right of self-defence may justify killing someone who knowingly threatens my life, it does not justify killing the innocent (i.e. someone who neither knows that they threaten my life nor intends to do so). How would Thomson respond to this criticism?

2. Consider this argument against Thomson: While it may be true that a woman is not obliged to save X's life by giving him the use of her body (or anything else for that matter), this does not mean that she has the right to kill X for using it. In the same way I am not obliged to save X's life by letting him use my home; but that does not mean that I have the right to kill him if I find him there. How would Thomson respond to this criticism? How would Noonan respond?

3. Do the duties of hospitality require that the mother must give birth to an unwanted baby?

4. In the light of the arguments presented by Purdy and Tooley, evaluate the claim that abortion should be available on demand.

5. A woman in labour will die unless an operation is performed in which the head of the unborn child is crushed or dissected. If it is not performed, the child can be successfully delivered by post-mortem Caesarean section. Construct arguments for and against these alternatives.

6. How do you account for the psychological fact that many persons who agree with abortion would shudder at the thought of murdering an innocent member of their own family.

7. Comment on the following statement: 'It is better for all the world, if instead of waiting to execute degenerate offspring for crime, or to let them starve for their imbecility, society can prevent those who are manifestly unfit from continuing their kind. The principle that sustains compulsory vaccination is broad enough to cover cutting the Fallopian tubes.' (Oliver Wendell Holmes)

8. What moral distinctions are to be drawn between abortion and contraception?

9. If a foetus has a right to life, does a defective foetus have a corresponding right not to be born?

10. Consider the following case. Assume you are the physician. What justification would you have for performing or not performing the abortion? What difference would it make if the foetus were defective?

A 35-year-old married woman, sixteen weeks pregnant, undergoes amniocentesis to determine the presence of foetal defects. The procedure, which takes about three weeks to complete, involves removing foetal cells from the fluid surrounding the foetus in the uterus, growing, and then analyzing the cells. The procedure carries little risk for either mother or child. Her physician reports that the foetus shows no sign of abnormality and that the woman can expect to give birth to a girl. Several days later the woman requests an abortion. The reason she gives the doctor is that she does not want to have another daughter. She has two children, 3 and 5 years old – both girls. Her husband is opposed to abortion and would prefer to have the additional child. The marriage appears to be stable and happy, and the couple are well-to-do. The physician did not know that the information regarding the sex of the foetus would lead to a request for an abortion.[10]

THE RIGHT TO LIFE AND EUTHANASIA

The right to life generates certain duties in others. Two in particular should be mentioned: the **duty of non-interference** and the **duty of service**. The duty of non-interference requires that no one should interfere in another's life in a way that may threaten it. So, if somebody is trying to shoot me, I have the right

10. *Ethics in Medicine*, edited by S J Reiser, A J Dyck and W J Curran, Cambridge, Mass.: The MIT Press, 1977, p.485.

to stop him. My right to life also allows me to claim certain duties from others, the duties of service, and these may be claimed of those who are in the business of seeing that my life is sustained (doctors, firemen, lifesavers). Both duties presuppose that being alive is in itself valuable and worth preserving, and that to save someone's life, or at least not to shorten it, is to benefit them. Normally this is true; but not always. Death from a bullet is probably preferable to death by starvation, and it is unlikely that a prisoner being tortured to death would accept a life-prolonging drug. Saving or prolonging someone's life is not therefore always to their advantage: in certain circumstances it might have been better if they had died earlier rather than later. Or, to put the matter another way, to say that someone has a right to life, while true, does not necessarily mean that exercising that right will bring them benefit or that those who safeguard it are their benefactors. What matters is the *quality* of their life and their *attitude* towards it, and both may challenge the duties of non-interference and service. For cases may arise in which not only should the duty of non-interference be withheld in the interests of certain individuals – their lives are deliberately terminated – but withheld by the very people who have a duty of service towards them.

Such cases introduce the problem of **euthanasia**. The original meaning of the word, derived from the Greek *eu* (good) and *thanasia* (death), is 'a quiet and easy death' as opposed to a violent or painful one. More recently it has come to mean 'the action of inducing a gentle and easy death' and so refers mainly to those actions, usually performed by a doctor, in which a person's life is deliberately terminated or shortened. These actions are also known as 'mercy killings' since the death involved must in some way end suffering and therefore be in the person's own interest. This altruistic concern distinguishes these cases from, say, the euthanasia programme introduced by Hitler in 1939 which gassed 275,000 people, mostly the physically or mentally sick and elderly. They were not killed to relieve their suffering but because they were no longer able to work.

These sinister possibilities continue to haunt discussions of euthanasia. Many believe that, once this form of killing is legalised, it will lead to others, to infanticide or euthanasia for the socially maladjusted or politically deviant. Others point to the risk of abuse by members of the family and by all those who stand to gain by the death of someone old or sick. For members of the medical profession the problems are more immediate and acute. Some doctors will have nothing to do with euthanasia, saying that their job is to save life and not to kill and pointing to the constant possibility of a wrong diagnosis or a new treatment. Others, meanwhile, have argued that, since medical science can prolong life almost indefinitely, what must now be protected is not so much a person's right to life but his *right to die*, and that to subject a patient to an unnaturally slow and often painful deterioration, simply because it is technically possible, is not only uncivilised and lacking in compassion for patient and family alike, but also an infringement of individual liberty.

This debate is further complicated by the fact that euthanasia applies to two different groups of person: those who can exercise their right to die and those who, because of their mental or physical condition, cannot. In the first group are all those who are terminally ill but mentally alert: since they know they are dying, often in acute pain, should they be allowed to die sooner rather than later? This group also includes those who are not terminally ill but have become, perhaps through some serious accident, totally paralysed or dependent on machines: they are not about to die and may suffer no pain, but they too are aware of their own deterioration. Should they be allowed to bring their suffering to an end? In the second group we find all those in irreversible coma, kept alive by a life-support machine, but for whom the technical definition of death as brain death does not apply. Here too are elderly people suffering from extreme senile dementia and new-born infants with incurable genetic defects. Since these people cannot exercise their right to die, should somebody else do so on their behalf? And if so, who?

Given the complexity of the issues involved here, and given that no two cases are the same, a simple theory of euthanasia, covering all eventualities, is impossible. Philosophers have, however, introduced a number of useful distinctions between types of euthanasia, which have been generally recognised if not universally accepted. The first is between voluntary and involuntary euthanasia. **Voluntary euthanasia** occurs when a mentally competent person requests their own death – many moralists argue that this is permissible since it is the equivalent of assisted suicide —whereas **involuntary euthanasia** applies to those who are unable to make this decision for themselves.

The second distinction is made between direct and indirect euthanasia, both referring to the method of inducing death. **Direct euthanasia** involves the use of something specific to cause it, and **indirect euthanasia** refers to those cases where death occurs as a side-effect of treatment (e.g. injecting a lethal dose of morphine to reduce pain).

The third distinction, which is the subject of James Rachels's essay, is between active and passive euthanasia. **Active euthanasia** is the same as direct euthanasia: it is the intentional act of mercy-killing; but **passive euthanasia** is not killing but letting die: it allows a person to die by withholding or stopping the treatment that sustains their life. Many doctors believe this is the most important distinction of all, and there is no doubt that passive euthanasia is often practised. Even the Roman Catholic Church accepts that letting patients die should sometimes be permitted. No one has the right to kill, says the Church, but equally no one is under an obligation to prolong life indefinitely. Rachels believes, however, that this much-exploited distinction is bogus and thus without moral significance. Active and passive euthanasia are one and the same thing. Therefore, if passive euthanasia is to be allowed, active euthanasia should be allowed as well.

This argument is challenged by Yale Kamisar in his response to another advocate of active euthanasia, Glanville Williams.[11] Williams' argument, like Rachels', although admittedly philosophically strong, fails when applied to everyday situations. Kamisar is sceptical, for example, about the doctor's ability to decide when a case is 'hopeless', and about the patient's ability to make a 'voluntary' decision. Additionally Kamisar highlights two legal objections. In

11. Williams, *The Sanctity of Life and the Criminal Law*, London, Faber and Faber, 1958.

the first place, any law allowing voluntary euthanasia is bound to be vague and so open to abuse. In order to protect the potential victims of such a law, Kamisar is thus willing to sacrifice those who 'in fact have no desire and no reason to linger on.' In the second place, a law allowing voluntary euthanasia is likely to lead to a law allowing involuntary euthanasia, to the legal right to kill the unwanted, and thus to a situation where the right to life can be withheld from those whom the state regards as nuisances. Voluntary euthanasia must therefore be rejected on the grounds that it is likely to lead us down a 'slippery slope', to a situation already familiar to us from the Nazi euthanasia programme, in which the law sanctions the murder of the incurable, senile, retarded, and racially inferior.

In the third extract, we move from philosophical and legal considerations of euthanasia to its actual implementation. Many physicians paradoxically support euthanasia but refuse to perform it themselves, arguing that to do so is contrary to their role as healers and preservers of life. This ethical dilemma is well illustrated in the much-publicised case of Dr Timothy Quill of Rochester, New York. In the following extract, Quill describes his assistance in the suicide of a leukemia patient, Diane. Although reported on the front page of the *New York Times* in 1991, no legal action was taken against him. Reactions to the case suggest that, in the public view, where such assistance is responsibly given, it is morally justifiable.

Extract 4: James Rachels: Active and Passive Euthanasia[12]

The distinction between active and passive euthanasia is thought to be crucial for medical ethics. The idea is that it is permissible, at least in some cases, to withhold treatment and allow a patient to die, but it is never permissible to take any direct action designed to kill the patient. This doctrine seems to be accepted by most doctors. . . . However, a strong case can be made against it. In what follows I will set out some of the relevant arguments, and urge doctors to consider this matter.

To begin with a familiar type of situation, a patient who is dying of incurable cancer of the throat is in terrible pain, which can no longer be satisfactorily stopped. He is certain to die within a few days, even if present treatment is continued, but he does not want to go on living for those days since the pain is unbearable. So he asks the doctor for an end to it, and his family joins in the request.

Suppose the doctor agrees to withhold treatment, as the conventional doctrine says he may. The justification for his doing so is that the patient is in terrible agony, and since he is going to die anyway, it would be wrong to prolong his suffering needlessly. But now notice this. If one simply withholds treatment, it may take the patient longer to die, and so he may suffer more than he would if more direct action were taken and a lethal injection given. This fact provides strong reason for thinking that, once the initial decision not to prolong his agony has been made, active euthanasia is actually preferable to passive euthanasia. To say otherwise is to endorse the option that leads to more suffering rather than less, and is contrary to the humanitarian impulse that prompts the decision not to prolong his life in the first place. . . .

One reason why so many people think that there is an important moral difference between active and passive euthanasia is that they think killing someone is

---

12. James Rachels, 'Active and Passive Euthanasia,' *New England Journal of Medicine*, 292 (1975). Reprinted in *Moral Problems*, ed. James Rachels, New York & London, Harper & Row, 1979, pp. 490-497.

morally worse than letting someone die. But is it? Is killing, in itself, worse than letting die? To investigate this issue, two cases may be considered that are exactly alike except that one involves killing whereas the other involves letting someone die. Then, it can be asked whether this difference makes any difference to the moral assessments. It is important that the cases be exactly alike, except for this one difference, since otherwise one cannot be confident that it is this difference and not some other that accounts for any variation in the assessments of the two cases. So, let us consider this pair of cases:

In the first, Smith stands to gain a large inheritance if anything should happen to his six-year old cousin. One evening while the child is taking his bath, Smith sneaks into the bathroom and drowns the child, and then arranges things so that it will look like an accident.

In the second, Jones also stands to gain if anything should happen to his six-year old cousin. Like Smith, Jones sneaks in planning to drown the child in his bath. However, just as he enters the bathroom Jones sees the child slip and hit his head, and fall face down in the water. Jones is delighted; he stands by, ready to push the child's head back under if it is necessary, but it is not necessary. With only a little thrashing about, the child drowns all by himself, as Jones watches and does nothing.

Now Smith killed the child, whereas Jones 'merely' let the child die. That is the only difference between them. Did either man behave better, from a moral point of view? If the difference between killing and letting die were in itself a morally important matter, one should say that Jones' behaviour was less reprehensible than Smith's. But does one really want to say that? I think not. In the first place, both men acted from the same motive, personal gain, and both had exactly the same end in view when they acted. It may be inferred from Smith's conduct that he is a bad man, although that judgement may be withdrawn or modified if certain further facts are learned about him – for example, that he is mentally deranged. But would not the very same thing be inferred about Jones from his conduct? And would not the same further considerations also be relevant to any modification of this judgement? Moreover, suppose Jones pleaded, in his own defense, 'After all, I didn't do anything except just stand there and watch the child drown. I didn't kill him; I only let him die.' Again, if letting die were in itself less bad than killing, this defense should have at least some weight. But it does not. Such a 'defense' can only be regarded as a grotesque perversion of moral reasoning. Morally speaking, it is no defense at all.

Now, it may be pointed out, quite properly, that the cases of euthanasia with which doctors are concerned are not like this at all. They do not involve personal gain or the destruction of normal healthy children. Doctors are concerned only with cases in which the patient's life is of no further use to him, or in which the patient's life has become or will soon become a terrible burden. However, the point is the same in these cases: the difference between killing and letting die does not, in itself, make a moral difference. If a doctor lets a patient die, for humane reasons, he is in the same moral position as if he had given the patient a lethal injection for humane reasons. If his decision was wrong – if, for example, the patients's illness was in fact curable – the decision would be equally regrettable no matter which method was used to carry it out. And if the doctor's decision was the right one, the method used is not in itself important. . . .

Many people will find this judgement hard to accept. One reason, I think, is that it is very easy to fuse the question of whether killing is, in itself, worse than letting die, with the very different question of whether most actual cases of killing are more reprehensible than most actual cases of letting die. Most actual cases of killing are clearly terrible (think, for example, of all the murders reported in the newspapers), and one hears of such cases every day. On the other hand, one hardly ever hears of a case of letting die, except for the actions of doctors who are motivated by humanitarian reasons. So one learns to think of killing in a much worse light than of letting die. But this does not mean that there is something about killing that makes it in itself worse than letting die, for it is not the bare difference between killing and letting die that makes the difference in these cases. Rather, the other factors – the murderer's motive of personal gain, for example, contrasted with the doctor's humanitarian motivation – account for different reactions to the different cases.

I have argued that killing is not in itself any worse than letting die; if my contention is right, it follows that active euthanasia is not any worse than passive euthanasia. What arguments can be given on the other side? The most common, I believe, is the following:

The important difference between active and passive euthanasia is that, in passive euthanasia, the doctor does not do anything to bring about the patient's death. The doctor does nothing, and the patient dies of whatever ills already afflict him. In active euthanasia, however, the doctor does something to bring about the patient's death: he kills him. The doctor who gives the patient with cancer a lethal injection has himself caused his patient's death; whereas if he merely ceases treatment, the cancer is the cause of death.

A number of points need to be made here. The first is that it is not exactly correct to say that in passive euthanasia the doctor does nothing, for he does do one thing that is very important: he lets the patient die. 'Letting someone die' is certainly different, in some respects, from other types of action – mainly in that it is a kind of action that one may perform by way of not performing certain other actions. For example, one may let a patient die by way of not giving medication, just as one may insult someone by way of not shaking his hand. But for any purpose of moral assessment, it is a type of action none the less. The decision to let a patient die is subject to moral appraisal in the same way that a decision to kill him would be subject to moral appraisal: it may be assessed as wise or unwise, compassionate or sadistic, right or wrong. If a doctor deliberately lets a patient die who was suffering from a routinely curable illness, the doctor would certainly be to blame for what he had done, just as he would be to blame if he had needlessly killed the patient.

Charges against him would then be appropriate. If so, it would be no defense at all for him to insist that he didn't 'do anything'. He would have done something very serious indeed, for he let his patient die.

Fixing the cause of death may be very important from a legal point of view, for it may determine whether criminal charges are brought against the doctor. But I do not think that this notion can be used to show a moral difference between active and passive euthanasia. The reason why it is considered bad to be the cause of someone's death is that death is regarded as a great evil – and so it is. However, if it has been decided that euthanasia – even passive euthanasia – is desirable in a given case, it has also been decided that in this instance death is no greater an evil than the patient's continued existence. And if this is true, the usual reason for not wanting to be the cause of someone's death simply does not apply.

Finally, doctors may think that all of this is only of academic interest – the sort of thing that philosophers may worry about but that has no practical bearing on their own work. After all, doctors, must be concerned about the legal consequences of what they do, and active euthanasia is clearly forbidden by the law. But even so, doctors should also be concerned with the fact that the law is forcing upon them a moral doctrine that may be indefensible, and has a considerable effect on their practices.

Extract 5: Yale Kamisar: Some Non-religious views against proposed 'Mercy-killing' legislation.[13]

As an ultimate philosophical proposition, the case for voluntary euthanasia is strong. Whatever may be said for and against suicide generally, the appeal of death is immeasurably greater when it is sought not for a poor reason or just reason, but for 'good cause,' so to speak; when it is invoked not on behalf of a 'socially useful' person, but on behalf of, for example, the pain-racked 'hopelessly incurable' cancer victim. If a person is *in fact* (1) presently incurable, (2) beyond the aid of any respite which may come along in his life expectancy, suffering (3) intolerable and (4) unmitigable pain and of a (5) fixed and (6) rational desire to die, I would hate to have to argue that the hand of death should be stayed. But abstract propositions and carefully formed hypotheticals are one thing; specific proposals designed to cover everyday situations are something else again.

In essence, Williams' specific proposal is that death be authorized for a person in the above situation 'by giving the medical practitioner a wide discretion and trusting to his good sense'. This, I submit, raises too great a risk of abuse and mistake to warrant a change in the existing law. That a proposal entails risk of mistake is hardly a conclusive reason against it. But neither is it irrelevant. Under any euthanasia program the consequences of mistake, of course, are always fatal. As I shall endeavor to show, the incidence of mistake of one kind or another is likely to be quite appreciable. If this indeed be the case, unless the need for the authorized conduct is compelling enough to override it, I take it the risk of mistake *is* a conclusive reason against such authorization. I submit too, that the possible radiations from the proposed legislations, e.g. involuntary euthanasia of idiots and imbeciles (the typical 'mercy-killings' reported by the press) and the emergence of the legal precedent that there are lives not 'worth living,' give additional cause to pause.

I see the issue, then, as the need for voluntary euthanasia versus (1) the incidence of mistake and abuse; and (2) the danger that legal machinery initially designed to kill those who are a nuisance to themselves may someday engulf those who are a nuisance to others. . . .

As will be seen, and as might be expected, the simple negative proposal to remove 'mercy-killings' from the ban of the criminal law is strenuously resisted on the ground that it offers the patient far too little protection from not-so-necessary or not-so-merciful killings. On the other hand, the elaborate affirmative proposals of the euthanasia societies meet much prolonged eye-blinking, not few guffaws, and sharp criticism that the legal machinery is so drawn-out, so complex, so formal and so tedious as to offer the patient far too little solace. . . .

It may just be, however, that . . . the trouble lies with the euthanasiasts themselves in seeking a goal which is *inherently inconsistent*: a procedure for death which *both* (1) provides ample safeguards against abuse and mistake; and (2) is 'quick and easy' in operation. . . . Evidently, the presumption is that the general practitioner is a sufficient buffer between the patient and the restless spouse or overwrought or overreaching relative, as well as a depository of enough general scientific know-how and enough information about current research developments and trends, to assure a minimum of error in diagnosis and anticipation of new measures of relief. Whether or not the general practitioner will accept the responsibility Williams would confer on him is itself a problem of major proportions. . . .

13. *Minnesota Law Review*, XLII, No. 6 (May, 1958), pp. 969-1042

Under current proposals to establish legal machinery, elaborate or otherwise, for the administration of a quick and easy death, it is not enough that those authorized to pass on the question decide that the patient, in effect, is 'better off dead.' The patient must concur in this opinion. Much of the appeal in the current proposal lies in this so-called 'voluntary' attribute.

But is the adult patient really in a position to concur? Is he truly able to make euthanasia a 'voluntary' act? There is a good deal to be said, is there not, for Dr Frohman's pithy comment that the 'voluntary' plan is supposed to be carried out 'only if the victim is both sane and crazed by pain.'[14] By hypothesis, voluntary euthanasia is not to be resorted to until narcotics have long since been administered and the patient has developed a tolerance to them. *When*, then, does the patient make the choice? While heavily drugged? Or is narcotic relief to be withdrawn for the time of decision? But if heavy dosages no longer deadens pain, indeed, no longer makes it bearable, how overwhelming is it when whatever relief narcotics offer is taken away, too?

Assuming, for purposes of argument, that the occasion when a euthanasia candidate possesses a sufficiently clear mind can be ascertained and that a request for euthanasia is then made, there remain other problems. . . . Even if the patient's choice could be said to be 'clear and incontrovertible,' do not other difficulties remain? Is this the kind of choice, assuming that it can be made in a fixed and rational manner, that we want to offer a gravely ill person? Will we not sweep up, in the process, some who are not really tired of life, but think others are tired of them; some who do not really want to die, but who feel they should live on, because to do so when there looms the legal alternative of euthanasia is to do a selfish and a cowardly act? Will not some feel an obligation to have themselves 'eliminated' in order that funds allocated for their terminal care might be better used by their families or, financial worries aside, in order to relieve their families of the emotional strain involved?

It would not be surprising for the gravely ill person to seek to inquire of those close to him whether he should avail himself of the legal alternative of euthanasia. Certainly, he is likely to wonder about their attitude in the matter. It is quite possible, is it not, that he will not exactly be gratified by any inclination of their part – however noble their motives may be in fact – that he resort to the new procedure? At this stage, the patient-family relationship may well be a good deal less than it ought to be. . . .

And what of the relatives? If their views will not always influence the patient, will they not at least influence the attending physician? Will a physician assume the risks to his reputation, if not his pocketbook, by administering the *coup de grace* over the objection – however irrational – of a close relative? Do not the relatives, then, also have a 'choice?' Is not the decision on their part to do nothing and say nothing *itself* a 'choice?' In many families there will be some, will there not, who will consider a stand against euthanasia the only proof of love, devotion and gratitude for past events? What of the stress and strife if close relatives differ . . . over the desirability of euthanatizing the patient? . . .

Faulty diagnosis is only one ground for error. Even if the diagnosis is correct, a second ground for error lies in the possibility that some measure of relief, if not a full cure, may come to the fore within the life expectancy of the patient. Since Glanville Williams does not deign this objection to euthanasia worth more than a passing reference, it is necessary to turn elsewhere to ascertain how it has been met.

One answer is:
It must be little comfort to a man slowly coming apart from multiple sclerosis to think that, fifteen years from now, death might not be his only hope.[15]

---

14. Frohman, *Vexing Problems in Forensic Medicine: A Physician's View*, 31 N. Y. U. L. Rev. 1215, 1222 (1956).

To state the problem this way is of course to avoid it entirely. How do we know that fifteen *days* or fifteen *hours* from now, 'death might not be [the incurable's] only hope?"

A second answer is:
[N]o cure for cancer which might be found 'tomorrow' would be of any value to a man or woman 'so far advanced in cancerous toxemia as to be an applicant for euthanasia'.

As I shall endeavor to show, this approach is a good deal easier to formulate that it is to apply. For one thing, it presumes that we know today *what* cures will be found tomorrow. For another, it overlooks that if such cases can be said to exist, the patient is likely to be *so far* advanced in cancerous toxemia as to be no longer capable of understanding the step he is taking and hence *beyond* the stage when euthanasia ought to be administered.

A generation ago, Dr Haven Emerson, then President of the American Public Health Association, made the point that 'no one can say today what will be incurable tomorrow. No one can predict what disease will be fatal or permanently incurable until medicine becomes stationary and sterile.' Dr Emerson went so far as to say that 'to be at all accurate we must drop altogether the term 'incurables' and substitute for it some such term as 'chronic illness".[16]

That was a generation ago. Dr Emerson did not have to go back more than a decade to document his contention. Before Banting and Best's insulin discovery, many a diabetic had been doomed. Before the Whipple-Minot-Murphy liver treatment made it a relatively minor malady, many a pernicious anemia sufferer had been branded 'hopeless.' Before the uses of sulfanilimide were disclosed, a patient with widespread streptococcal blood poisoning was a condemned man.

Today, we may take even that most resolute disease, cancer, and we need look no further than the last decade of research in this field to document the same contention. . . . True, many types of cancer still run their course virtually unhampered by man's arduous efforts to inhibit them. But the number of cancers coming under some control is ever increasing. With medicine attacking on so many fronts with so many weapons who would bet a man's life on when and how the next type of cancer will yield, if only just a bit?

True, we are not betting much of a life. For even in those areas where gains have been registered, the life is not 'saved', death is only postponed. Of course, in a sense this is the case with every 'cure' for every ailment. But it may be urged that after all there is a great deal of difference between the typical 'cure' which achieves an indefinite postponement, more or less, and the cancer respite which results in only a brief intermission, so to speak, of rarely more than six months or a year. Is this really long enough to warrant all the bother?

Well, how long *is* long enough? In many recent cases of cancer respite, the patient, though experiencing only temporary relief, underwent sufficient improvement to retake his place in society. Six or twelve or eighteen months is long enough to do most of the things which socially justify our existence, is it not? Long enough for a nurse to care for more patients, a teacher to impart learning to more classes, a judge to write a great opinion, a novelist to write a stimulating book, a scientist to make an important discovery and, after all, for a factory hand to put the wheels on another year's Cadillac. . . .

(There) is the 'wedge principle,' the 'parade of horrors' objection, if you will, to voluntary euthanasia. . . . It is true that the 'wedge' objection can always be advanced, the horrors can always be paraded. But it is no less true that on some occasions the objection is much more valid than it is on others. One reason why

15. 'Pro and Con: Shall be Legalize "Mercy Killing"?' *Readers Digest*, November, 1938, pp.94, 96.
16. 'Who is Incurable? A Query and Reply". *New York Times*, October 22, 1933, p.5.

the 'parade of horrors' cannot be too lightly dismissed in this particular instance is that Miss Voluntary Euthanasia is not likely to be going it alone for very long. Many of her admirers. . . . would be neither surprised nor distressed to see her joined by Miss Euthanatize the Congenital Idiots and Miss Euthanatize the Permanently Insane and Miss Euthanatize the Senile Dementia. And these lasses – whether or not they themselves constitute a 'parade of horrors' – certainly make excellent majorettes for such a parade. . . .

Another reason why the 'parade of horrors' argument cannot be too lightly dismissed in this particular instance, it seems to me, is that the parade *has* taken place in our own time and the order of procession has been headed by the killing of the 'incurables' and the 'useless'. . . .

It may be conceded that in a narrow sense it is an 'evil' for . . . a patient to have to continue to suffer – if only for a little while. But in a narrow sense, long-term sentences and capital punishment are 'evils', too. If we can justify the infliction of imprisonment and death by the state 'on the ground of the social interests to be protected'[17], then surely we can similarly justify the postponement of death by the state. The objection that the individual is thereby treated not as an 'end' in himself but only as a 'means' to further the common good was, I think, aptly disposed of by Holmes long ago. 'If a man lives in society, he is likely to find himself so treated.'[18].

Extract 6:   Timothy Quill: Death and Dignity[19]

Diane was feeling tired and had a rash. A common scenario, though there was something subliminally worrisome that prompted me to check her blood count. Her hematocrit was 22, and the white-cell count was 4.3 with some metamyelocytes and unusual white cells. I wanted it to be viral, trying to deny what was staring me in the face. Perhaps in a repeated count it would disappear. I called Diane and told her it might be more serious than I had initially thought – that the test needed to be repeated and that if she felt worse, we might have to move quickly. When she pressed for the possibilities, I reluctantly opened the door to leukemia. Hearing the word seemed to make it exist. 'Oh, shit!' she said. 'Don't tell me that.' Oh, shit! I thought, I wish I didn't have to.

Diane was no ordinary person (although no one I have ever come to know has been really ordinary). She was raised in an alcoholic family and had felt alone for much of her life. She had vaginal cancer as a young woman. Through much of her adult life, she had struggled with depression and her own alcoholism. I had come to know, respect, and admire her over the previous eight years as she confronted these problems and gradually overcame them. She was an incredibly clear, at times brutally honest, thinker and communicator. As she took control of her life, she developed a strong sense of independence and confidence. In the previous 3 years, her hard work had paid off. She was completely abstinent from alcohol, she had established much deeper connections with her husband, college-age son, and several friends, and her business and her artistic work were blossoming. She felt she was really living fully for the first time.

Not surprisingly, the repeated blood count was abnormal, and detailed examination of the peripheral-blood smear showed myelocytes. I advised her to come into the hospital, explaining that we needed to do a bone marrow biopsy and make some decisions relatively rapidly. She came to the hospital knowing what we would find. She was terrified, angry, and sad. Although we knew the odds, we both clung to the thread of possibility that it might be something else.

The bone marrow confirmed the worst: acute myelomonocytic leukemia. In

17. *Crime, Law and Social Science*, 351, (1933)
18 *The Common Law*, 44, (1881)
19. *The New England Journal of Medicine*, vol. 324, No. 10 (March 7, 1991), pp. 691-694.

the face of this tragedy, we looked for signs of hope. This is an area of medicine in which technological intervention has been successful, with cures 25 percent of the time – long-term cures. As I probed the costs of these cures, I heard about induction chemotherapy (three weeks in the hospital, prolonged neutropenia, probable infectious complications, and hair loss; 75 percent of patients respond, 25 percent do not). For the survivors, this is followed by consolidation chemotherapy (with similar side effects; another 25 percent die, for a net survival of 50 percent). Those still alive, to have a reasonable chance of long-term survival, then need bone marrow transplantation (hospitalization for two months and whole-body irradiation, with complete killing of the bone marrow, infectious complications, and the possibility of graft-versus-host disease – with a survival of approximately 50 percent, or 25 percent of the original group). Though hematologists may argue over the exact percentages, they don't argue about the outcome of no treatment – certain death in days, weeks, or at most a few months.

Believing that delay was dangerous, our oncologist broke the news to Diane and began making plans to insert a Hickman catheter and begin induction chemotherapy that afternoon. When I saw her shortly thereafter, she was enraged at his presumption that she would want treatment, and devastated by the finality of the diagnosis. All she wanted to do was go home and be with her family. She had no further questions about treatment and in fact had decided that she wanted none. Together we lamented her tragedy and the unfairness of life. Before she left, I felt the need to be sure that she and her husband understood that there was some risk in delay, that the problem was not going to go away, and that we needed to keep considering the options over the next several days. We agreed to meet in two days.

She returned in two days with her husband and son. They had talked extensively about the problem and the options. She remained very clear about her wish not to undergo chemotherapy and to live whatever time she had left outside the hospital. As we explored her thinking further, it became clear that she was convinced she would die during the period of treatment and would suffer unspeakably in the process (from hospitalization, from lack of control over her body, from the side effects of chemotherapy, and from pain and anguish). Although I could offer support and my best effort to minimize her suffering if she chose treatment, there was no way I could say any of this would not occur. In fact, the last four patients with acute leukemia at our hospital had died very painful deaths in the hospital during various stages of treatment (a fact I did not share with her). Her family wished she would choose treatment but sadly accepted her decision. She articulated very clearly that it was she who would be experiencing all the side effects of treatment and that odds of 25 percent were not good enough for her to undergo so toxic a course of therapy, given her expectations of chemotherapy and hospitalization and the absence of a closely matched bone marrow donor. I had her repeat her understanding of the treatment, the odds, and what to expect if there were no treatment. I clarified a few misunderstandings, but she had a remarkable grasp of the options and implications.

I have been a longtime advocate of active, informed patient choice of treatment or nontreatment, and of a patient's right to die with as much control and dignity as possible. Yet there was something about her giving up a 25 percent chance of long-term survival in favor of almost certain death that disturbed me. I had seen Diane fight and use her considerable inner resources to overcome alcoholism and depression, and I half expected her to change her mind over the next week. Since the window of time in which effective treatment can be initiated is rather narrow, we met several times that week. We obtained a second hematology consultation and talked at length about the meaning and implications of treatment and nontreatment.

She talked to a psychologist she had seen in the past. I gradually understood the decision from her perspective and became convinced that it was the right decision for her. We arranged for home hospice care (although at that time Diane felt reasonably well, was active, and looked healthy), left the door open for her to change her mind, and tried to anticipate how to keep her comfortable in the time she had left.

Just as I was adjusting to her decision, she opened up another area that would stretch me profoundly. It was extraordinarily important to Diane to maintain control of herself and her own dignity during the time remaining to her. When this was no longer possible, she clearly wanted to die. As a former director of a hospice program, I know how to use pain medicines to keep patients comfortable and lessen suffering. I explained the philosophy of comfort care, which I strongly believe in. Although Diane understood and appreciated this, she had known of people lingering in what was called relative comfort, and she wanted no part of it. When the time came, she wanted to take her life in the least painful way possible. Knowing of her desire for independence and her decision to stay in control, I thought this request made perfect sense. I acknowledged and explored this wish but also thought that it was out of the realm of currently accepted medical practice and that it was more than I could offer or promise. In our discussion, it became clear that preoccupation with her fear of a lingering death would interfere with Diane's getting the most out of the time she had left until she found a safe way to ensure her death. I feared the effects of a violent death on her family, the consequences of an ineffective suicide that would leave her lingering in precisely the state she dreaded so much, and the possibility that a family member would be forced to assist her, with all the legal and personal repercussions that would follow. She discussed this at length with her family. They believed that they should respect her choice. With this in mind, I told Diane that information was available from the Hemlock Society that might be helpful to her.

A week later she phoned me with a request for barbiturates for sleep. Since I knew that this was an essential ingredient in a Hemlock Society suicide, I asked her to come to the office to talk things over. She was more than willing to protect me by participating in a superficial conversation about her insomnia, but it was important to me to know how she planned to use the drugs and to be sure that she was not in despair or overwhelmed in a way that might color her judgment. In our discussion, it was apparent that she was having trouble sleeping, but it was also evident that the security of having enough barbiturates available to commit suicide when and if the time came would leave her secure enough to live fully and concentrate on the present. It was clear that she was not despondent and that in fact she was making deep, personal connections with her family and close friends. I made sure that she knew how to use the barbiturates for sleep, and also that she knew the amount needed to commit suicide. We agreed to meet regularly, and she promised to meet with me before taking her life, to ensure that all other avenues had been exhausted. I wrote the prescription with an uneasy feeling about the boundaries I was exploring – spiritual, legal, professional, and personal. Yet I also felt strongly that I was setting her free to get the most out of the time she had left, and to maintain dignity and control on her own terms until her death.

The next several months were very intense and important for Diane. Her son stayed home from college, and they were able to be with one another and say much that had not been said earlier. Her husband did his work at home so that he and Diane could spend more time together. She spent her time with her closest friends. I had her come into the hospital for a conference with our residents, at which she illustrated in a most profound and personal way the importance of informed decision making, the right to refuse treatment, and the extraordinarily personal effects of illness and interaction with the medical system. There were emotional and physical hardships as well. She had periods of intense sadness and anger. Several times she became very weak, but she received transfusions as an outpatient and responded with marked improvement of symptoms. She had two serious infections that responded surprisingly well to empirical courses of oral antibiotics. After three tumultuous months, there were two weeks of relative calm and well-being, and fantasies of a miracle began to surface.

Unfortunately, we had no miracle. Bone pain, weakness, fatigue, and fevers began to dominate her life. Although the hospice workers, family members, and I tried our best to minimize the suffering and promote comfort, it was clear that the end was approaching. Diane's immediate future held what she feared most – increasing discomfort, dependence, and hard choices between pain and sedation. She called up her closest friends and asked them to come over to say goodbye, telling them that she would be leaving soon. As we had agreed, she let me know as well. When we met, it was clear that she knew what she was doing, that she was sad and frightened to be leaving, but that she would be even more terrified to stay and suffer. In our tearful goodbye, she promised a reunion in the future at her favorite spot on the edge of Lake Geneva, with dragons swimming in the sunset.

Two days later her husband called to say that Diane had died. She had said her final goodbyes to her husband and son that morning, and asked them to leave her alone for an hour. After an hour, which must have seemed an eternity, they found her on the couch, lying very still and covered by her favorite shawl. There was no sign of struggle. She seemed to be at peace. They called me for advice about how to proceed. When I arrived at their house, Diane indeed seemed peaceful. Her husband and son were quiet. We talked about what a remarkable person she had been. They seemed to have no doubts about the course she had chosen or about their cooperation, although the unfairness of her illness and the finality of her death were overwhelming to us all.

I called the medical examiner to inform him that a hospice patient had died. When asked about the cause of death, I said, 'acute leukemia.' He said that was fine and that we should call a funeral director. Although acute leukemia was the truth, it was not the whole story. Yet any mention of suicide would have given rise to a police investigation and probably brought the arrival of an ambulance crew for resuscitation. Diane would have become a 'coroner's case,' and the decision to perform an autopsy would have been made at the discretion of the medical examiner. The family or I could have been subject to criminal prosecution, and I to professional review, for our roles in support of Diane's choices. Although I truly believe that the family and I gave her the best care possible, allowing her to define her limits and directions as much as possible, I am not sure the law, society, or the medical profession would agree. So I said 'acute leukemia' to protect all of us, to protect Diane from an invasion into her past and her body, and to continue to shield society from the knowledge of the degree of suffering that people often undergo in the process of dying. Suffering can be lessened to some extent, but in no way eliminated or made benign, by the careful intervention of a competent, caring physician, given current social constraints.

Diane taught me about the range of help I can provide if I know people well and if I allow them to say what they really want. She taught me about life, death, honesty and about taking charge and facing tragedy squarely when it strikes. She taught me that I can take small risks for people that I really know and care about. Although I did not assist in her suicide directly, I helped indirectly to make it possible, successful, and relatively painless. Although I know we have measures to help control pain and lessen suffering, to think that people do not suffer in the process of dying is an illusion. Prolonged dying can occasionally be peaceful, but more often the role of the physician and family is limited to lessening but not eliminating severe suffering.

I wonder how many families and physicians secretly help patients over the edge into death in the face of such severe suffering. I wonder how many severely ill or dying patients secretly take their lives, dying alone in despair. I wonder whether the image of Diane's final aloneness will persist in the minds of her family, or if they will remember more the intense, meaningful months they had together before she died. I wonder whether Diane struggled in that last hour, and whether the Hemlock Society's way of death by suicide is the most benign. I wonder why Diane, who gave so much to so many of us, had to be alone for the last hour of her life. I wonder whether I will see Diane again, on the shore of Lake Geneva at sunset, with dragons swimming on the horizon.

Questions: Euthanasia

1. Analyse the teleological character of Rachels's argument? How might a deontologist reply?

2. What is the difference between active and passive euthanasia? Do you think this difference is morally justified? What are its practical implications for the medical profession?

3. Assess Kamisar's 'slippery slope' argument. What dangers can you foresee in the legalization of euthanasia, and how might they be overcome?

4. Was Timothy Quill right to do what he did? Defend your position against possible objections.

5. 'No human being should be allowed to exist in a state which we would mercifully end in any other creature.' Discuss.

6. Do people have the right to commit suicide? If they have this right, should the state provide them with the means to achieve it?

7. 'If physicians have a license to kill, they will forever lose the trust and respect of their patients.' Discuss.

8. What parallels are to be drawn between objections to euthanasia and objections to capital punishment?

9. Is euthanasia justified on the grounds that it directs limited resources away from so-called 'futile' cases? Should a distinction be made here between insured and uninsured patients?

10. Consider the following case:

> The third night that I roomed with Jack in our tiny double room in the solid-tumor ward of the cancer clinic of the National Institutes of Health in Bethesda, Md., a terrible thought occurred to me.
> Jack had a melanoma in his belly, a malignant solid tumor that the doc-

tors guessed was about the size of a softball. The cancer had started a few months before with a small tumor in his left shoulder, and there had been several operations since. The doctors planned to remove the softball-sized tumor, but they knew Jack would soon die. The cancer had metastasized – it had spread beyond control.

Jack was good-looking, about 28, and brave. He was in constant pain, and his doctor had prescribed an intravenous shot of a synthetic opiate – a pain-killer, or analgesic – every four hours. His wife spent many of the daylight hours with him, and she would sit or lie on his bed and pat him all over, as one pats a child, only more methodically, and this seemed to help control the pain. But at night, when his pretty wife had left (wives cannot stay overnight at the NIH clinic) and darkness fell, the pain would attack without pity.

At the prescribed hour, a nurse would give Jack a shot of the synthetic analgesic, and this would control the pain for perhaps two hours or a bit more. Then he would begin to moan, or whimper, very low, as though he didn't want to wake me. Then he would begin to howl, like a dog.

When this happened, either he or I would ring for a nurse, and ask for a pain-killer. She would give him some codeine or the like by mouth, but it never did any real good – it affected him no more than half an aspirin might affect a man who had just broken his arm. Always the nurse would explain as encouragingly as she could that there was not long to go before the next intravenous shot – 'Only about 50 minutes now.' And always poor Jack's whimpers and howls would become more loud and frequent until at last the blessed relief came.

The third night of this routine, the terrible thought occurred to me. 'If Jack were a dog,' I thought, 'what would be done with him?' The answer was obvious: the pound, and chloroform. No human being with a spark of pity could let a living thing suffer so, to no good end.[20]

Bibliography: The Right to Life

* denotes text extracted in main text

1) The Right to Life and Abortion

Batchelor, Edward (ed.) *Abortion: The Moral Issues*, New York, The Pilgrim Press, 1982. A general anthology.

Berkowitz, Jonathan 'How I was almost aborted: reflections on a prenatal brush with death,' *Journal of Medical Ethics*, xvii, 1991, pp.136-137.

Feinberg, Joel (ed.) *The Problem of Abortion*, Belmont, Calif: Wadsworth, 1973. Contains Thomson's essay and Michael Tooley's important article, 'A Defense of Abortion and Infanticide'.

Glover, Jonathan *Causing Death and Saving Lives*, Harmondsworth, 1977.

Harris, John *The Value of Life*, Routledge & Kegan Paul, 1985. Extensive discussion, with chapters on abortion and euthanasia.

Hursthouse, Rosalind *Beginning Lives*, Oxford: Basil Blackwell, in association with the Open University, 1987.

Noonan, John T 'How to Argue about Abortion,'* reprinted in *Contemporary Issues in Bioethics*, edited, with Introductions, by Tom L Beauchamp and

20. Stewart Alsop, 'The Right to Die With Dignity,' *Good Housekeeping*, August 1974, pp. 69, 130.

LeRoy Walters, Dickenson Publishing Company, Encino, Calif., 1978, pp.210-217.

Perkins, Robert (ed.) *Abortion. Pro and Con*, Cambridge, Mass: 1974. Anthology.

Purdy, Laura, and Michael Tooley. 'Is Abortion Murder?'* in *Abortion: Pro and Con*, ed. by Robert L. Perkins, Cambridge, Mass., Schenkman, 1974, pp.129-136.

Reiser, S J (ed. with A J Dyck and W J Curran). *Ethics in Medicine*, Cambridge, Mass: The MIT Press, 1977.

Sumner, L W *Abortion and Moral Theory*, Princeton, NJ: Princeton University Press, 1981. Argues that both the liberal and conservative views are indefensible.

Thomson, Judith Jarvis *Rights, Restitution and Risk*,* ed. William Parent, Cambridge, Mass: Harvard University Press, 1986. A collection of Thomson's essays, the first being her famous article on abortion.

Tooley, Michael *Abortion and Infanticide*, Oxford: Clarendon Press, 1983. One of the most influential liberal discussions.

2) The Right to Life and Euthanasia

Anon 'It's Over, Debbie,' *Journal of the American Medical Association*, vol. 259, 1988, pp.272, 2094-98, 2139-2143. A famous anonymous article, which provoked a storm of controversy.

Behnke, John A and Bok, Sissela *The Dilemmas of Euthanasia*, Garden City, NY: Anchor Books, 1975. An excellent anthology.

Dominica, Frances 'Reflections on death in childhood,' *British Medical Journal*, vol. 294, January 1987, pp.108-110. A moving account of hospice care.

Downing, A E (ed.) *Euthanasia and the Right to Death*, London: 1969. Essays arguing for voluntary euthanasia.

Foot, Philippa 'Euthanasia,' in *Medicine and Moral Philosophy*, edited by Marshall Cohen, Thomas Nagel, Thomas Scanlon, Princeton, N.J., Princeton, 1981, pp.276-303.

Gorovitz, S, Janeton, A L et al (eds) *Moral Problems in Medicine*, Englewood Cliffs, NJ, Prentice-Hall, 1976. Excellent anthology.

Gould, Jonathan (ed. with Lord Craigmyle) *Your Death Warrant?* London, Chapman, 1971. Essays against euthanasia.

Horan, Dennis J (ed. with David Mall) *Death, Dying and Euthanasia*, Frederick, Maryland, University Publications of America, 1980. Thorough anthology.

Kamisar, Yale. 'Some non-religious views against proposed "Mercy-killing" legislation',* *Minnesota Law Review*, XLII, No.6 (May, 1958) pp.969-1042

Kohl, Marvin (ed.) *Beneficent Euthanasia*, Buffalo, NY: Prometheus Books, 1975. Wide-ranging anthology.

Kubler-Ross, Elizabeth. *On Death and Dying*, New York: Macmillan, 1974. A distinguished psychiatrist on the attitudes of the terminally ill.

Ladd, John (ed.) *Ethical Issues Relating to Life and Death*, Oxford, Oxford University Press, 1979. A collection of philosophical discussions.

Quill, Timothy E 'Death and Dignity: A Case of Individualized Decision Making', * *The New England Journal of Medicine*, vol.324, No.10, March 7, 1991, pp.691-694.

Ramsey, Paul *Ethics at the Edges of Life*, Pt 2, New Haven, Conn: Yale University Press, 1978. A stimulating, if difficult, analysis by a leading contemporary moralist.

Rachels, James 'Active and Passive Euthanasia',* *New England Journal of Medicine*, 292 (1975). Reprinted in *Moral Problems*, ed James Rachels, New York & London: Harper & Row, 1979) pp. 490-497.

Saunders, Cicely 'The Last Stages of Life,' *American Journal of Nursing*, vol.65, No.3, 1965, pp.70-75. Written by a pioneer of hospice care.

Supreme Court of New Jersey. *In the Matter of Karen Quinlan. An Alleged Incompetent*, decided March 31, 1976, Supreme Court of New Jersey 355A 2nd 647. Reprinted in *Killing and Letting Die*, ed Bonnie Steinbeck, Englewood NJ: Prentice-Hall, 1980, pp 23-44. Perhaps the most famous case of involuntary euthanasia.

Williams, Robert H. *To Live and To Die: When, Why, and How?* New York, Springer-Verlag, (1973) A wide-ranging anthology.

Chapter Four
Utilitarianism

THE THEORY OF JEREMY BENTHAM

Egoism, in as much as it calculates what we ought to do in terms of an action's consequences, is a straightforward teleological theory of moral behaviour. Its weakness, as we have seen, lies primarily in the fact that it appears to take no account of the effects of such an action on other people, particularly on those who, for various reasons, cannot adequately defend themselves. In the previous chapter we saw how this pursuit of an egoistic philosophy raised serious moral questions: in the debate about abortion, for example, we were led to consider whether the right to life should be extended to the unborn, and, in the debate about euthanasia, whether this right should, in quite specific circumstances, be denied to those still living.

This weakness of egoism can, however, be fairly easily overcome in another ethical and teleological theory, to which we shall now turn. This maintains that it is the *total* consequences of an action which determines its rightness or wrongness; that, in other words, it is not just my happiness or self-interest which counts but the happiness or self-interest of everyone concerned. This is the theory known as **utilitarianism**. Utilitarianism states that *an action is right if it produces the greatest good for the greatest number.*

The two greatest advocates of utilitarianism are Jeremy Bentham (1748-1832) and his disciple John Stuart Mill (1806-1873). While it is true that Mill gives the most famous 'proof' of utilitarianism, it is to Bentham that we must first turn as the theory's chief exponent and populariser.

Jeremy Bentham was a man of extraordinary intellectual gifts: at three years old he began to study Latin, at five French, and, in 1763, he took his degree at Oxford at the age of sixteen. Given these abilities, and the fact that both his father and grandfather were attorneys, a great legal career was predicted for him. However, five years later, while reading Priestley's *Essay on Government*, he came upon the expression 'the greatest good of the greatest number', and says that he cried out, like Archimedes, 'Eureka'. Bentham decided to apply this principle, which he called the **principle of utility**, to all areas of social activity and thereby to do for human society what Newton had done for natural science.

Bentham's chief interest was 'legislation', for it is the legislator, he maintained, who alone has the power of determining the conditions under which men live. In his great work, the *Principles of Morals and Legislation* (1789) he impressed on his contemporaries the belief that existing institutions were not to be taken for granted but critically judged by their *effects* or *consequences*, and so reformed as to produce the 'greatest good of the greatest number.' This procedure extended across the whole range of social life and initiated a series of reforms for which Bentham was either directly or indirectly responsible: the reform of the representative system of Parliament and the drafting of its Acts; the reform of the criminal law, the jury system, and prisons; the abolition of transportation and imprisonment for debt; the development of saving banks, cheap postage, and the registration of births and deaths. As if this were not enough, he was probably the first man to suggest the Suez and Panama canals and the formation of a League of Nations. Following his belief that the dead should be of some use to the living, he left his body to be dissected in the presence of friends. His skeleton was then reconstructed, clothed in Bentham's usual attire, and set upright in a glass-fronted case: it is now kept in University College, London.

THE PRINCIPLE OF UTILITY

From this brief sketch of Bentham's life we can see the clear teleological character of the utilitarian argument. Just as we judge a law or an institution in terms of its effect on the majority of citizens, so the morality of our own actions is to be judged in terms of their effect on all concerned, i.e. whether they do or do not lead to the greatest happiness for the greatest number. According to Bentham, therefore, the correct ethical standard is the **principle of utility**, the word 'utility' referring to the tendency of something to produce happiness, not to its usefulness.

> By the principle of utility is meant that principle which approves or disapproves of every action whatsoever, according to the tendency which it appears to have to augment or diminish the happiness of the party whose interest is in question: or, what is the same thing in other words, to promote or to oppose that happiness. I say of every action whatsoever; and therefore not only of every action of a private individual, but of every measure of government[1]

The principle of utility states, therefore, that an action ought to be done if and only if it brings about the maximum possible happiness for those parties affected by that action. But what counts as an 'affected party'? Even though it is quite possible to treat a state of community as an affected party – after all, we can speak of crimes against the state or of serving the community – it is quite clear that Bentham is here talking of individuals. For him 'state', 'community', 'nation' are nothing more than collective terms denoting groups of individuals. One cannot, therefore, speak of the 'state' over against those persons who compose it. Accordingly, the principle of utility refers only to individual actions by individuals, its simple message being that the more happiness produced by these actions the better the world will be. These actions must of course be voluntary because the very idea of moral responsibility depends on the person concerned having a real choice of whether to perform the action or not.

But how does one choose? If an immediate action (A) produces less happiness than an action in the future (B), I should perform B rather than A. However, in deciding between A and B, I must also take account of the possible

---

1. *An Introduction to the Principles of Morals and Legislation*, ed. J H Burn and H L A Hart, London & New York, Methuen, 1982, p.12.

unhappiness resulting from them. If A produces less happiness but also less unhappiness than B, then B's greater unhappiness detracts from its greater happiness. Thus I must choose A if thereby a greater *sum total* of happiness is produced. If, on the other hand, *both* A and B produce the same amounts of happiness, but B more unhappiness, I must still choose A. By this action I produce the greatest balance of happiness over unhappiness.

This explains why, when there is a choice between 1) greater happiness for myself, and 2) less happiness for myself and greater happiness for others, I must choose the latter. My greater happiness cannot take precedence over the greatest *net* happiness, i.e. the happiness of all those involved. It is of course quite possible that one action will produce both my greatest happiness *and* the greatest total happiness; but when there is a conflict of interest – when my happiness conflicts with the greater collective happiness – then utilitarianism advises self-sacrifice, even to the point of death. Needless to say, in such extreme circumstances, it is all the more important to be convinced that one's calculations are correct.

In making these calculations, however, another feature of Bentham's theory should be noted. Bentham was a **hedonist** and thus believed, like Epicurus before him, that pleasure was the sole good and pain the sole evil. This is clearly stated in the opening sentences of the *Principles of Morals and Legislation:*

> Nature has placed mankind under the governance of two sovereign masters, pain and pleasure. It is for them alone to point out what we ought to do, as well as to determine what we shall do. On the one hand the standard of right and wrong, on the other the chain of causes and effects, are fastened to their throne. They govern us in all we do, in all we say, in all we think: every effort we can make to throw off our subjection, will serve but to demonstrate and confirm it. In words a man may pretend to abjure their empire: but in reality he will remain subject to it all the while. The principle of utility recognises this subjection, and assumes it for the foundation of that system, the object of which is to rear the fabric of felicity by the hands of reason and of law. Systems which attempt to question it, deal in sounds instead of sense, in caprice instead of reason, in darkness instead of light.[2]

More exactly, then, it is the twin experiences of pleasure and pain which govern the operation of the principle of utility: it is the fact of these experiences that determines what we ought and ought not to do. If we generally accept, for example, that such things as honesty, affection and mercy are characteristics of the moral life, this is not because, to use an earlier terminology, they have any **intrinsic** value (i.e. that they are pleasurable in themselves), but because they have an **instrumental** value (i.e. that these are qualities that lead to pleasure). If, on the other hand, these things did not have this effect – if they brought us misery instead – then we would not credit them with any moral value. For Bentham, an act is right only when it is instrumentally good; and its goodness consists in the pleasure produced. Thus the moral worth of one action over against another is directly proportional to the amount or quality of pleasure

2. *Ibid.*, p.11.

(or pain) that each action brings. This being the case, a more accurate account of the principle of utility would read: *For all those affected by an action, that action is right if it brings pleasure (or prevents pain), and wrong if it brings pain (or prevents pleasure.)*

THE HEDONIC CALCULUS

As soon as we state the principle of utility in this new form, another problem immediately arises. If, in our calculation of what we ought to do, we must take into account the possible pleasure or pain involved for everyone (including the agent), then how do we assess or estimate the quantity of pleasure and pain involved? How, for instance, do we gauge whether this pleasure is greater than another, or whether this particular pain outweighs that particular pleasure? It is in order to help us in these calculations that Bentham introduces his **hedonic calculus**.

Bentham's hedonic calculus turns on the idea that human pleasures and pains are measurable, and that accordingly actions can be judged right or wrong on the basis of a kind of 'moral arithmetic', the sums involved corresponding to the amount of pleasure or pain these actions contain. Bentham is quite ready to admit that the experience of pleasure is unusually complex, that few pleasures are completely 'pure', and that most have a fair measure of pain mixed up with them. Nor does he minimise the difficulty in trying to calculate the amount of pleasure found, say, in wealth as against power or in the use of one's skill as against one's imagination; but all these factors are, he says, accounted for in the calculus and quantifiable in terms of the seven *circumstances* or *dimensions* in which pleasure occurs:

> To a person considered by **himself**, the value of a pleasure or pain considered by itself, will be greater or less, according to the four following circumstances:
> 1. Its **intensity**
> 2. Its **duration**
> 3. Its **certainty** or **uncertainty**
> 4. Its **propinquity** or **remoteness**
>
> These are the circumstances which are to be considered in estimating a pleasure or a pain. But when the value of any pleasure or pain is considered for the purpose of estimating the tendency of any act by which it is produced, there are two other circumstances to be taken into the account:
>
> 5. Its **fecundity**, or the chance it has of being followed by sensations of the same kind: that is, pleasures, if it be a pleasure: pains, if it be a pain.
> 6. Its **purity**, or the chance it has of **not** being followed by sensations of the opposite kind: that is, pains, if it be a pleasure; pleasures, if it be a pain.
>
> These last two, however, are in strictness scarcely to be deemed properties of the pleasure or the pain itself; they are not, therefore, in strictness to be taken into the account of the value of that pleasure or that pain. They are in strictness to be deemed properties only of the act, or other event, by which

such pleasure or pain has been produced; and accordingly are only to be taken into the account of the tendency of such act or such event.

To a **number** of persons, with reference to each of whom the value of a pleasure or a pain is considered, it will be greater or less, according to seven circumstances: to wit, the six preceding ones . . . and one other; to wit:

7. Its **extent**; that is, the number of persons to whom it extends; or (in other words) who are affected by it.[3]

To see how this calculus works, let us suppose that you are a poor man badly in need of a drink. An acquaintance of yours, whom you know to be rich, passes you in the street and accidentally drops his wallet. You pick it up and inside find £50. Should you return it to him? You decide by consulting the hedonic calculus. Various factors can be dismissed immediately: *extent*, because clearly only the two of you are involved; and *certainty* and *propinquity*, because, in this case, there is little doubt that both of you will experience some pleasure and some pain, and that these experiences will be near in time to the actual moment when you picked up the wallet. On the other hand, if you do decide to keep the money, one factor will almost certainly count against you – *purity* – because it is highly probable that your pleasure will also contain some pain (i.e. a feeling of guilt at taking the money, a possible hangover from taking the drink). Nevertheless, even these possibilities will not detract from the *overall* balance of pleasure in your favour. It is, for example, a fair bet that your pleasure at finding the money will be more *intense* than the rich man's irritation at its loss; that your pleasure will *last longer* than his pain; and that your pleasure will produce other pleasures in a way that his initial pain will not produce other pains – indeed, being rich, he will probably quickly forget all about it. On these calculations, it is clear that you should keep the money. You could, of course, return the money; but even then it is unlikely that the rich man's pleasure at its recovery will equal your pain at its loss.

---

3. *Ibid.*, pp. 38-39. In order to popularise his hedonic calculus and to give it more general appeal, Bentham composed the following memoriter verses:

Intense, long, certain, speedy, fruitful, pure -
Such marks in *pleasures* and in *pains* endure.
Such pleasures seek if *private* be thy end:
If it be *public*, wide let them *extend*.
Such *pains* avoid, whichever be they view:
If pains *must* come, let them *extend* to few.

Exercise 1

In which of the following situations would you adopt utilitarian principles? Explain your answers.

1. Should a doctor be permitted to administer a drug that will painlessly kill a person with an incurable disease? Would it make any difference to your opinion if that patient were your rich father?

2. Should contraceptives be provided free of charge to the unmarried?

3. Should the governments of overpopulated countries close down all fertility clinics?

4. Are there any cases in which sterilization should be carried out without the patient's consent?

5. Given its limited resources, should a hospital always give priority to the treatment of the young over the old?

6. Should a baby's life be saved for a future of suffering: hospitals, drugs, operations?

7. A priest hears the confession of a married man, who is HIV. Should the priest inform the man's wife?

8. If statistics prove that smoking is bad for your health, should the government outlaw smoking?

9. If my mother is happier in a private clinic than in a public ward, does this justify private health care?

10. Mother Teresa, Louis Pasteur and Joe Bloggs (an ex-convict) are in a boat. The boat is sinking. Who should drown to save the other two?

Questions: Bentham

1. One objection to Bentham's theory is that it can be used to justify immoral actions. Do you agree? How do you think Bentham would reply to this criticism?

2. Should Bentham's principle of utility extend to animals? What would the consequences be if it did?

3. Is the utility of an action the only morally significant factor? Would it therefore be right for me to refuse to pay my mother's hospital bills on the grounds that I can make better use of the money?

4. Following Bentham's example, are all of us morally obligated to donate our bodies to medical research?

5. In the following passage, the contemporary philosopher Ayn Rand objects to Bentham's formula, 'the greatest good of the greatest number.' What are the grounds of her objection? Do you agree with her?

'The good of others' is a magic formula that transforms anything into gold . . . your code hands out, as its version of the absolute, the following rule of moral conduct: if you wish it, it's evil; if others wish it, it's good; if the motive of your action is your welfare, don't do it; if the motive is the welfare of others, anything goes. . . . For those of you who might ask questions, your code provides a consolation prize and a booby trap: it is your own happiness, it says, that you serve the happiness of others, the only way to achieve your joy is to give it up to others . . . and if you find no joy in this procedure, it is your own fault and the proof of your evil . . . a morality that teaches you to scorn a whore who gives her body indiscriminately to all men – this same morality demands that you surrender your soul to promiscuous love for all comers.[4]

THE THEORY OF JOHN STUART MILL

For Bentham there can be no moral rules other than those ordained by the principle of utility. As we saw in the previous case of finding £50, this often means that the consequences of a so-called 'immoral' act – stealing, lying, breaking promises, killing – are preferable to those of the alternative so-called 'moral' act. This does not mean that Bentham rejects all the rules of conventional morality, since he is quite ready to accept that, in most cases, they serve to increase human happiness; but these rules, he maintains, must never be followed blindly. When taking ethical decisions, we should be guided by the principle of utility and not by the rules of social custom or convention.

All this seems quite straightforward. Most of us would agree that, while stealing is in general wrong, it would be right to steal a weapon from a homicidal maniac. Similarly, we say that lying is wrong but would approve, say, of someone giving false information to an enemy agent. Common sense, and an overall desire to increase the sum total of human happiness, dictate that we would be justified in doing these things. Bentham's theory gets into difficulties when it condones actions which, even though increasing the total amount of pleasure, are still held to be *morally inexcusable*. Suppose that a group of sadistic guards are torturing a prisoner. If the guards' pleasure outweighs the prisoner's pain, then, according to the hedonic calculus, their action is justified. Indeed, we soon see that the calculus may be used to support any number of morally repugnant acts. It will, for example, justify any majority of persons suppressing the human rights of any minority. If the majority receives happiness because a small minority are slaves, it will support slavery. This does not of course imply that Bentham would have approved of slavery, sadism or genocide; but they do lead us to reject a principle which may be used to justify such repugnant acts.

This does not mean, however, that we have found a sufficient reason for rejecting utilitarianism altogether, if only because Bentham presents only one particular version of the theory. Another is proposed by his disciple and friend,

---

4. *Atlas Shrugged*, New York, Random House, 1957, p.1030-1033.

John Stuart Mill. Mill's version is an explicit attempt to meet the kind of objection just raised.

At first sight Mill's theory does not appear to be very different from Bentham's. Like his predecessor, Mill is a hedonist, believing that pleasure is the sole intrinsic good, and that it is the promotion of pleasure and the prevention of pain that determines our moral decisions. Thereafter, however, the difference between the two theories is considerable, and appears primarily when Mill rejects Bentham's purely **quantitative** assessment of pleasure and replaces it with a **qualitative** one. Mill puts far greater stress on the variety of pleasures and distinguishes between their respective values. He maintains that some pleasures, namely those of the mind, are higher and more estimable than others, namely, those of the body. With this new version of utilitarianism, Mill believed that he could defend the doctrine against the kind of attack earlier levelled against Bentham. It is now possible to say, for instance, that the pleasure experienced by the sadistic guards does not justify their actions because this particular kind of pleasure is of so low a value that it does not outweigh the acute pain experienced by the prisoner. Mill describes his position in the following extract from his essay, *Utilitarianism* (1863):

Mill: The Greatest Happiness Principle[5]

The creed which accepts as the foundation of morals Utility, or the Greatest Happiness Principle, holds that actions are right in proportion as they tend to promote happiness, wrong as they tend to produce the reverse of happiness. By 'happiness' is intended pleasure, and the absence of pain; by 'unhappiness', pain, and the privation of pleasure. To give a clear view of the moral standard set up by the theory, much more requires to be said; in particular, what things it includes in the ideas of pain and pleasure; and to what extent this is left an open question. But these supplementary explanations do not affect the theory of life on which this theory of morality is grounded – namely, that pleasure, and freedom from pain, are the only things desirable as ends; and that all desirable things (which are as numerous in the utilitarian as in any other scheme) are desirable either for the pleasure inherent in themselves, or as means to the promotion of pleasure and the prevention of pain.

Now such a theory of life excites in many minds, and among them in some of the most estimable in feeling and purpose, inveterate dislike. To suppose that life has (as they express it) no higher end than pleasure, no better and nobler object of desire and pursuit, they designate as utterly mean and grovelling; as a doctrine worthy only of swine, to whom the followers of Epicurus were, at a very early period, contemptuously likened; and modern holders of the doctrine are occasionally made the subject of equally polite comparisons by its German, French, and English assailants.

When thus attacked, the Epicureans have always answered that it is not they, but their accusers, who represent human nature in a degrading light; since the accusation supposes human beings to be capable of no pleasures except those of which swine are capable. If this supposition were true, the charge could not be gainsaid, but would then be no longer an imputation: for if the sources of pleasure were precisely the same to human beings and to swine, the rule of life which is good enough for the

---

5. Reprinted in *Utilitarianism, Liberty, and Representative Government,* with an introduction by A D Lindsay, London, J M Dent & Sons, 1948, pp.6-11.

one would be good enough for the other. The comparison of the Epicurean life to that of beasts is felt as degrading, precisely because a beast's pleasures do not satisfy a human being's conceptions of happiness. Human beings have faculties more elevated than the animal appetites, and when once made conscious of them, do not regard anything as happiness which does not include their gratification . . . But there is no known Epicurean theory of life which does not assign to the pleasure of the intellect, of the feelings and imagination, and of the moral sentiments, a much higher value as pleasures than those of mere sensation . . . It is quite compatible with the principle of utility to recognize the fact, that some *kinds* of pleasure are more desirable and more valuable than others. It would be absurd that while, in estimating all other things, quality is considered as well as quantity, the estimation of pleasures should be supposed to depend on quantity alone.

If I am asked what I mean by difference of quality in pleasures, or what makes one pleasure more valuable than another, merely as a pleasure, except its being greater in amount, there is but one possible answer. Of two pleasures, if there be one to which all or almost all who have experience of both give a decided preference, irrespective of any feeling of moral obligation to prefer it, that is the more desirable pleasure. If one of the two is, by those who are competently acquainted with both, placed so far above the other that they prefer it, even though knowing it to be attended with a greater amount of discontent, and would not resign it for any quantity of the other pleasure which their nature is capable of, we are justified in ascribing to the preferred enjoyment a superiority in quality, so far outweighing quantity as to render it, in comparison, of small account.

Now it is an unquestionable fact that those who are equally acquainted with, and equally capable of appreciating and enjoying, both, do give a most marked preference to the manner of existence which employs their higher faculties. Few human creatures would consent to be changed into any of the lower animals, for a promise of the fullest allowance of a beast's pleasures; no intelligent human being would consent to be a fool, no instructed person would be an ignoramus, no person of feeling and conscience would be selfish and base, even though they should be persuaded that the fool, the dunce, or the rascal is better satisfied with his lot than they are with theirs. They would not resign what they possess more than he, for the most complete satisfaction of all the desires which they have in common with him. If they ever fancy they would, it is only in cases of unhappiness so extreme, that to escape from it they would exchange their lot for almost any other, however undesirable in their own eyes. A being of higher faculties requires more to make him happy, is capable probably of more acute suffering, and certainly accessible to it at more points, than one of an inferior type; but in spite of these liabilities, he can never really wish to sink into what he feels to be a lower grade of existence . . . It is better to be a human being dissatisfied than a pig satisfied; better to be Socrates dissatisfied than a fool satisfied. And if the fool, or the pig, is of a different opinion, it is because they only know their own side of the question. The other party to the comparison knows both sides.

It may be objected, that many who are capable of the higher pleasures, occasionally, under the influence of temptation, postpone them to the lower. But this is quite compatible with a full appreciation of the intrinsic superiority of the higher. Men often, from infirmity of character, make their election for the nearer good, though they know it to be the less valuable; and this no less when the choice is between two bodily pleasures, than when it is between bodily and mental. They pursue sensual indulgences to the injury of health, though perfectly aware that health is the greater good. It may be further objected, that many who begin with youthful enthusiasm for everything noble, as they advance in years sink into indolence and selfishness. But I do not believe that those who undergo this very common change, voluntarily choose the lower description of pleasures in preference to the higher. I believe that before they devote themselves exclusively to the one, they have already become incapable of the other. Capacity for the nobler feelings is in most natures a very tender plant, easily killed, not only by hostile influences, but by mere want of sustenance; and in the majority of young persons it speedily dies away if the occupations to which their position in life has devoted them, and the society into which it has thrown them, are not favourable to keeping that higher capacity in exercise. Men lose their higher aspirations as they lose their intellectual tastes, because they have not time or opportunity for indulging them; and they addict themselves to inferior pleasures, not because they deliberately prefer them, but because they are either the only ones to which they have access, or the only ones which they are any longer capable of enjoying. It may be questioned whether anyone who has remained equally susceptible to both classes of pleasures, ever knowingly and calmly preferred the lower; though many, in all ages, have broken down in an ineffectual attempt to combine both.

From this verdict of the only competent judges, I apprehend there can be no appeal. On a question which is the best worth having of two pleasures, or which of two modes of existence is the most grateful to the feelings, apart from its moral attributes and from its consequences, the judgement of those who are qualified by knowledge of both, or, if they differ, that of the majority among them, must be admitted as final. And there needs be the less hesitation to accept this judgement respecting the quality of pleasures, since there is no other tribunal to be referred to even on the question of quantity. What means are there of determining which is the acutest of two pains; or the intensest of two pleasurable sensations, except the general suffrage of those who are familiar with both? Neither pains nor pleasures are homogeneous, and pain is always heterogeneous with pleasure. What is there to decide whether a particular pleasure is worth purchasing at the cost of a particular pain, except the feelings and judgement of the experienced? When, therefore, those feelings and judgement declare the pleasures derived from the higher faculties to be preferable in kind, apart from the question of intensity, to those of which the animal nature, disjoined from the higher faculties, is susceptible, they are entitled on this subject to the same regard.

I have dwelt on this point, as being a necessary part of a perfectly just conception of Utility, or Happiness, considered as the directive rule of human conduct. But it is by no means an indispensable condition to the acceptance of the utilitarian standard; for that standard is not the agent's own greatest happiness, but the greatest amount of happiness altogether; and if it may possibly be doubted whether a noble character is always the happier for its nobleness, there can be no doubt that it makes other people happier, and that the world in general is immensely a gainer by it. Utilitarianism, therefore, could only attain its end by the general cultivation of nobleness of character, even if each individual were only benefited by the nobleness of others, and his own, so far as happiness is concerned, were a sheer deduction from the benefit. But the bare enunciation of such an absurdity as this last, renders refutation superfluous.

Exercise 2

Which of the following do you consider 'higher' or 'lower' pleasures? List both sets of pleasures in an order of preference – counting +10 and - 10 for maximum and minimum pleasure – and then compare your list with other people's. Have you come to a majority view? Has Mill's distinction proved useful or not?

A		B	
a.	Having money	a.	Forgiving your enemies
b.	Having power	b.	Drinking champagne
c.	Having friends	c.	Drinking water
d.	Saying your prayers	d.	Playing football
e.	Eating pork	e.	Playing chess
f.	Giving love	f.	Playing an instrument
g.	Receiving love	g.	Listening to Mozart
h.	Making love	h.	Going to a rock concert
i.	Taking a walk	i.	Reading poetry
j.	Taking revenge	j.	Writing poetry

Questions: Mill

1. Do you think an intellectual's life is qualitatively superior to that of a fool?

2. What are the social implications of Mill's theory?

3. Why is there a conflict between Bentham's utilitarianism and justice? Illustrate your answer with a specific example. Does Mill overcome this conflict?

4. How successful is Mill's defence against the charge that utilitarianism is a 'swine ethic'?

5. How would you distinguish between the music of Mozart and the Beatles? Would you say that one involves a 'higher' art than the other?

6. Consider the following passage taken from Mill's *On Liberty* (1859). Here Mill argues that a person's expressed desires may be interfered with when these desires will do him harm. Does this argument justify health care professionals overriding the wishes of patients? Give examples.

> If either a public officer or any one else saw a person attempting to cross a bridge which had been ascertained to be unsafe, and there was no time to warn him of his danger, they might seize him and turn him back, without any real infringement of his liberty; for liberty consists in doing what one desires, and he does not desire to fall into the river.[6]

6. *On Liberty*, edited by David Spitz, New York, W W Norton & Co., 1975, p.89

SOME CRITICISMS OF UTILITARIANISM

In substituting quality for quantity, Mill's version of utilitarianism differs radically from Bentham's. Mill rejects a quantitative estimate of pleasure because, he argues, human beings, while experiencing 'lower' pleasures in common with the animals – i.e. the pleasures of food, drink, sex etc – are capable of certain other 'higher' pleasures – those of the intellect – which are beyond the reach of all other sentient beings. This difference between the 'higher' and 'lower' pleasures is, says Mill, sufficient to establish the distinctive range and variety of human happiness, and the unique character of man's pursuit of it in his moral life.

But how do we distinguish between these two orders of pleasure? People's opinions as to what are the higher and lower pleasures differ widely, and it is difficult to see how any general agreement could ever be reached. Mill answers by appealing to what he calls the 'competent judges'. If we want to know which are the higher and lower pleasures, then we must appeal to those who have experienced *both* kinds of pleasure. If these judges consistently opt for one pleasure over another, no matter how much pain or discomfort may accompany it, then this pleasure must be qualitatively superior. An opinion poll amongst these judges would reveal that they consistently choose the pleasures of the intellect in preference to the so-called 'lower' pleasures. As Mill remarked, ' . . . it is an unquestionable fact that those who are equally capable of appreciating and enjoying (both kinds of pleasure), do give a marked preference to the manner of existence which employs their higher faculties.'

This is all very well; but is it really an unquestionable fact that these so-called competent judges would always decide in favour of the higher pleasures? Certainly there is no *logical* reason why they should. Doubtless Mill would think it inconceivable for an intelligent Victorian gentleman to prefer the lower pleasures; but inconceivable though it may be to Mill, it is not for that reason impossible. Cases abound in which a man has thought an action pleasurable even though his society has regarded it with distaste; but this alone does not make it *wrong*. Majority opinion, even among the most educated, cannot, in other words, make a particular action *morally right* any more than it can make a scientific theory *empirically true*. The fact that the majority of citizens in ancient Rome approved of slavery does not justify their having slaves.

There are, however, other objections to utilitarianism, to which both Mill's version and Bentham's are equally exposed. Three in particular should be mentioned:-

The Problem of Consequences

If the rightness of an action depends on it producing the greatest balance of happiness over unhappiness, of pleasure over pain, then making a moral decision involves calculating that action's effects. But how is it possible to calculate all the possible consequences of an action? How can we ever be sure that any action will produce the greatest net happiness? We might be able to say, with some certainty, that this action (A) will have this consequence (B) in five minutes time; but B will inevitably have other consequences, and these consequences will in turn have other effects, and so on, until the end of time. At what point, therefore, do we make our calculations and determine that our original action was right or wrong?

The Problem of Special Responsibilities

Most of us accept that we have special responsibilities to particular people; we further accept that the rightness of these responsibilities does not necessarily derive from the fact that they increase the sum total of human happiness. This, however, is precisely what the utilitarian does not appear to admit. If, to use an earlier example, two men are drowning, and one is your father and the other a famous scientist on the verge of curing cancer, the utilitarian would urge you to save the scientist. Many of us would disagree and find such a suggestion repugnant. We would reply that we have a special duty towards our parents that outweighs any claim that a stranger, however illustrious, may have upon us. Other examples can be given. A teacher has a special obligation to his pupils; and despite what his pupils may think, this does not necessarily involve giving maximum marks in order to maximise the overall happiness of the class concerned. Indeed, in these cases, it is not unknown that an increase in quality is effected by an increase in pain. Thus it is that a teacher may discharge his duty without regard to the principle of utility.

The Problem of Justice

It may seem strange that justice should be a problem for utilitarianism. After all, the theory does correct the apparent 'selfishness' of ethical egoism, and it does insist that, when we calculate the effects of an action, no one person can claim special privileges and set aside the happiness of others in the pursuit of their own. Utilitarianism does seek to be *impartial*, and this we might think is necessary to any meaningful idea of justice – as indeed it is. But in another sense utilitarianism is not specifically egalitarian. For while we are told to aim for the greatest possible amount of happiness, and to count everybody's happiness equally, we are not told how this happiness is to be distributed. What happens, for instance, in those cases where the greatest amount of happiness is achieved but through an *unequal* distribution; in which, say, one person is deprived of happiness altogether? One such case involves the punishment of an innocent person. If we assume, as Bentham does, that the main aim of punishment is deterrence (making people obey the law through fear of what will happen to them if they don't), then a utilitarian judge would be right to condemn someone to death, knowing that they were innocent, if he believed that a greater good would result – such as restoring law and order, preventing an increase in crime, and so on. The problem is, that while this action may well maximise the sum total of happiness, it may yet be regarded as unjust in the way this sum is distributed. *For justice also demands dealing with individuals according to their deserts or merits.* On this reasoning, people are not punished because of what they may do or because of the effects of their punishment on others, but solely because of what they themselves have or have not done. If it is shown that no offence was committed, then their innocence is *alone* sufficient to justify their acquittal.

This conclusion is extremely significant. If justice is not necessarily served by the principle of utility, if the production of the greatest happiness does not imply that justice has been done, then we must conclude that deciding what is right and wrong requires more than a mere analysis of effects. We must move, that is, away from teleological theories and towards those which consider the extent to which the morality of an act depends on the nature of the act itself. In a word, we must begin to think **deontologically**.

Questions: Utilitarianism

1. In the Roald Dahl story 'Genesis and Catastrophe', a doctor saves both mother and child in a difficult birth.[7] His concluding words are, 'You'll be alright now, Mrs Hitler.' To what extent is this story a justified criticism of utilitarianism?

2. Give examples of what you consider to be the higher and lower pleasures. What problems does the difference between them present for deciding between right and wrong actions?

3. Justify the use of drugs to **(a)** alleviate physical pain, **(b)** reduce stress, and **(c)** induce a state of well-being.

4. Is it a valid criticism of utilitarianism that is permits medical experiments on the helpless?

5. Consider the following case. Does it represent a justified criticism of utilitarianism? How would a utilitarian reply?

Jim finds himself in the central square of a small South American town. Tied up against the wall are a row of twenty Indians, most terrified, a few defiant, in front of them several armed men in uniform. A heavy man in a sweat-stained khaki shirt turns out to be the captain in charge and, after a good deal of questioning of Jim which establishes that he got there by accident while on a botanical expedition, explains that the Indians are a random group of the inhabitants who, after recent acts of protest against the government, are just about to be killed to remind other possible protesters of the advantages of not protesting. However, since Jim is an honoured visitor from another land, the captain is happy to offer him a

7. *Kiss Kiss*, Harmondsworth, Penguin, 1962, pp.156-163.

guest's privilege of killing one of the Indians himself. If Jim accepts, then as a special mark of the occasion, the other Indians will be let off. Of course, if Jim refuses, then there is no special occasion, and Pedro here will do what he was about to do when Jim arrived, and kill them all. Jim, with some desperate recollection of schoolboy fiction, wonders whether if he got hold of a gun, he could hold the captain, and the rest of the soldiers to threat, but it is quite clear from the set-up that nothing of that kind is going to work: any attempt at that sort of thing will mean that all the Indians will be killed, and himself. The men against the wall, and the other villagers, understand the situation, and are obviously begging him to accept. What should he do?[8]

Bibliography: Utilitarianism

* denotes text extracted in main text.

Bayles, Michael D (ed.) *Contemporary Utilitarianism*, Garden City, N.Y., Doubleday, 1968. Collection of essays by contemporary philosophers.

Bentham, Jeremy *An Introduction to the Principles of Morals and Legislation,** edited by J H Burns and H L A Hart, London & New York, Methuen, 1982.

Gorovitz, Samuel (ed.) *John Stuart Mill: Utilitarianism with Critical Essays*, Indianapolis, Bobbs-Merrill, 1971.

Mill, John Stuart 'Utilitarianism,'* in *Utilitarianism, Liberty, and Representative Government*, with an Introduction by A D Lindsay, London, J M Dent & Sons, 1948.

Plamenatz, J *The English Utilitarians*, Oxford, Basil Blackwell, 1966. Chapter 4 on Bentham, Chapter 6 on Mill.

Quinton, Anthony *Utilitarian Ethics*, London, Gerald Duckworth, 1989. Excellent short introduction, with chapters on Bentham, Mill, and their critics.

Smart, J J C, with Bernard Williams. *Utilitarianism: For and Against,** Cambridge, Cambridge University Press, 1973. A defence and criticism of utilitarianism by two contemporary philosophers.

Sen, Amartya, and Bernard Williams (eds.) *Utilitarianism and Beyond*, Cambridge, Cambridge University Press, 1982. A wide range of arguments for and against.

Sprigge, T L S *The Rational Foundation of Ethics*, London and New York, Routledge & Kegan Paul, 1988. Especially Chapter 1. Chapter 2 contains an equally useful account of Moore and Ross.

---

8. Bernard Williams, *Utilitarianism: For and Against,* Cambridge, Cambridge University Press, 1973, pp. 98-99.

Chapter Five

Discussion: Utilitarianism and the Ethics of Experimentation

HUMAN EXPERIMENTATION

We must now consider how utilitarianism deals with certain medical-ethical problems. Because utilitarianism is a **teleological** theory of ethics, it will come as no surprise to discover that utilitarian health professionals tend to concern themselves with the consequences of any particular medical decision and judge whether their decisions are good or bad according to the principle of utility, that is, whether they do or do not increase the sum total of human happiness. We remember also that both Bentham and Mill were **hedonists**, and that both their quantitative and qualitative calculations were thus based on the assumption that happiness involves pleasure and the absence of pain and that unhappiness involves pain and the absence of pleasure. As Mill made clear, 'pleasure, and freedom from pain, are the only things desirable as ends.'[1] It is primarily this equation which determines how the utilitarian will resolve a medical dilemma. We know, for example, that many surgical procedures involve pain, and that accordingly they must be viewed as **intrinsic evils**. However, they may equally be viewed as **instrumental goods** if the pain inflicted brings a greater and long-term benefit to the patient or, applying the hedonic category of extent, to all those who might additionally benefit. Sometimes, of course, the choice can be an agonizing one for both patient and doctor alike. The decision, after all, may not be clear-cut. In a previous extract,[2] Dr Quill's patient, Diane, decided that the pain and indignity to be endured in the treatment of her leukemia outweighed the pleasure to be gained by prolonging her life. This was a utilitarian calculation on her part: her suicide not only removed her own pain but also removed the burden of care from her family and the possibility of legal action against them if they assisted in her death. Her decision, in other words, was not purely egoistic because it took account of the possible effects that her action would have on others.

We may express this utilitarian position by returning to the two duties mentioned earlier when discussing the right to life: the duty of non-interference and the duty of service.[3] In normal circumstances we reject as morally outrageous the right of anyone to endanger our right to life through their interference; and we also expect that certain groups of people (e.g. doctors, the police) will see to it that, whenever possible, that right to life is protected and sustained. But this may not always be the case. Situations may arise in which we request interference from the very people who have the duty of service towards us. Thus it is that health professionals are often asked to override their duties of service and perform abortions or withhold treatment from the terminally ill. Again, from the utilitarian viewpoint, their actions will be morally justified if, in the calculation

1. See above, p. 67
2. See above, p 53.
3. See above, p 44.

of happiness, a greater overall balance of pleasure over pain is achieved. The following three extracts expose some of the problems resulting from this position.

In the first section of this chapter we consider the application of utilitarian ethics to the question of human experimentation. In discussing this issue it is usual to distinguish between experimentation and therapy. The aim of therapy is to benefit an individual or group. This can be achieved, for example, through the diagnosis, treatment or prevention of a disease. Experimentation, by contrast, has as its aim the acquisition of new knowledge, most clearly seen in the testing of new drugs under controlled laboratory conditions. In practice, however, this distinction is not always so straightforward. An experiment can itself be therapeutic if, while its primary intention remains to serve the patient, it also aims to secure new information (e.g. the effectiveness of AZT in the treatment of AIDS). An experiment can also be non-therapeutic if no patient benefit is intended (e.g. the infection of healthy patients with the common cold).

The question is: Is human experimentation ever justified? The utilitarian response is predictably teleological: experiments of this kind bring extensive social benefit, and stopping them would bring corresponding harm. If the principle of our moral action is therefore to procure the greatest good for the greatest number, then a human volunteer participating in studies of antibiotics (like penicillin) or vaccines (like the polio vaccine) is acting in a moral way: he is contributing to the sum total of human happiness, even if no happiness accrues to him. The problem with this is that the same argument holds if participation in the experiment is not voluntary. The utilitarian justification remains in place notwithstanding the fact that the individual has been coerced into an experiment or remains ignorant of what is happening to him. It can still be argued that, like generals commanding soldiers to risk death in wartime, researchers need not seek permission from their human subjects in their battle against disease.

It is this aspect of human experimentation which concerns us most of all, not least because we are haunted by the memory of the Nazi experiments. As has often been pointed out, the philosophical justification for these atrocities was invariably utilitarian. The mass extermination of the chronically sick was justified on the grounds of saving 'useless' expenses to the rest of the community, and the mass extermination of Jews and gypsies justified because they were racially and socially unfit. A utilitarian ethic was also employed in the Nazi medico-military programme. Prisoners were shot to study gunshot wounds, live dissections were undertaken to show the effects of explosive decompression, and because it was known that soldiers did not long survive immersion in the North Sea, experiments on shock from exposure to cold were conducted at Dachau and Auschwitz.[4] But these atrocities are not peculiar to concentration camps. It is also worth recalling that, in Alabama from 1932 to 1972, the United States Public Health Service funded the Tuskeegee Study, which was set up to investigate the effects of untreated syphilis on 400 black males. Notoriously these subjects knew neither the precise nature of their disease nor the fact that it was treatable with penicillin.[5] In this instance the desire to

4. See Leo Alexander, 'Medical Science under Dictatorship', *The New England Journal of Medicine*, 241, No. 2, 14 July, 1949, pp. 39-47.
5. See James Jones, *Bad Blood*, New York, Free Press, 1981. A useful account of the case is given by Gregory E Pence, *Classic Cases in Medical Ethics*, New York,McGraw-Hill, 1990, pp. 184-203.

resolve an experimental question – 'Is the treatment of syphilis with a new drug more effective than no treatment at all?' – resulted in withholding altogether the therapeutic concern for the patient. In May 1997 President Clinton formally apologised for the abuses incurred during this programme. Other notorious examples of illicit experimentation are not difficult to find. Often cited is the research undertaken at Willowbank State School on Staten Island (1956), which involved the deliberate infection of retarded children with hepatitis, the cancer programme at the Jewish Chronic Disease Hospital (1963), which involved the injection of live cancer cells into patients, and, much more recently, the testing of unapproved drugs on military personnel during the Gulf War (1991).

In the first extract which follows, the theologian Paul Ramsey proposes a deontological safeguard against these illicit utilitarian justifications of human experimentation. This safeguard is the principle of informed consent, which he calls the cardinal 'canon of loyalty' to which both doctor and patient must be subject. This right to consent is, he argues, an inalienable right, and thus any research project which denies this right is using a person as a means rather than an end. Ramsey admits there may be difficulties in upholding this principle – the patient, after all, may lack the technical competence to make a judgment in the matter; but he claims that it is a necessary principle, highlighting the patient's role as a 'co-adventurer' in the battle against disease. The requirement of consent makes clear that, however laudable the utilitarian aim to obtain the greatest possible benefit for others, this aim cannot justify the exploitation of the individual for the advantage of others. This principle of consent, of course, provides no safeguard to those from whom consent cannot be sought. What, for example, of cases involving children, the mentally defective, the insane, the unconscious, and those requiring emergency surgery? Ramsey has argued that, because the 'canon of loyalty' cannot apply in these instances, no experimentation should be undertaken unless of direct benefit to the patient. But what, then, of those cases in which no benefit can accrue to the subject? What, for example, of those cases involving the unborn and the dead?

In the second extract George J Annas provides a detailed analysis of one such case, and here too he questions the benefits of the experiment and whether proper consent was obtained. This is the famous case of Baby Fae, a five-pound baby girl born on 12 October, 1984. She was diagnosed as having a hypoplastic left heart syndrome, a condition in which the left side of the heart is underdeveloped and thus unable to pump blood. Life expectancy is a matter of weeks. In an operation known as a xenograft, the chief of pediatric surgery at Loma Linda Hospital, Dr Leonard Bailey, replaced Baby Fae's heart with that of a baboon. Twenty days later Baby Fae died.

Given Bentham's strong views about the use of the dead for the benefit of the living, and his own donation of his body for dissection, there is little doubt that he would thoroughly approve of many of the proposals made Willard Gaylin in our third extract. Because no happiness can accrue to the dead, it is easy to suppose that the utilitarian concern for the living should be paramount. Gaylin therefore depicts a society in which the wholesale and systematic salvage of useful body parts is made possible by new technology. He proposes the development of special hospitals or banks or farms of cadavers, which could then be 'harvested' for organ donation and experimentation. Although cost-effective and of enormous educational significance, the fact, however, that many of us will view such a scheme with horror may indicate, says Gaylin, a legitimate refusal to reduce ourselves to the level of expendable matter.

Extract 1: Paul Ramsey: The Ethics of Consent[6]

One need not read very far in medical ethics – and especially not in the literature concerning medical experimentation or the ethical 'codes' that have been formulated since the medical cases at the Nuremberg trials – without realizing that medical ethics has not its sole basis in the overall benefits to be produced. It is not a consequence-ethics alone. It is not solely a teleological ethics, to use the language of philosophy. It is not even an ethics of the 'greatest possible medical benefits for the greatest possible number' of people. That calculus too easily comes to mean the 'greatest possible medical benefits regardless of the number' of patients who without their proper consent may be made the subjects of promising medical investigations. Medical ethics is not solely a benefit-producing ethics even in regard to the individual patient, since he should not always be helped without his will.

As stated in the *Ethical Guidelines for Organ Transplantation* of the American Medical Association[7], so also of medical experimentation involving human subjects: 'Man participates in these procedures: he is the patient in them; or he performs them. All mankind in the ultimate beneficiary of them.' Observe that the respect in which man is the patient and man the performer of medical care or medical investigation (the relation between doctor and patient/subject) places an independent moral limit upon the fashion in which the rest of mankind can be made the ultimate beneficiary of these procedures. In the language of philosophy, a deontological dimension or test holds chief place in medical ethics, beside teleological considerations. That is to say, there must be a determination of the rightness or wrongness of the action and not only of the good to be obtained in medical care or from medical investigation.

A crucial element in answer to the question, What constitutes right action in medical practice? is the requirement of a reasonably free and adequately informed consent. In current medical ethics, this is the chief *canon of loyalty* (as I shall call it) between the man who is patient/subject and the man who performs medical investigational procedures. Physicians discuss the consent-requirement just as ethicists discuss fairness- or justice-claims: these tests must be satisfied along with the benefits (the 'good') obtained. . . .

The principle of an informed consent is a statement of the fidelity between the man who performs medical procedures and the man on whom they are performed. Other aspects of medical ethics – for example, the requirement of a good experimental design and of professional skill at least as good as is customary in ordinary medical practice – treat the man as a purely passive subject or patient. These are also the requirements that hold for an ethical experiment upon animals. But any human being is more than a patient or experimental subject; he is a *personal* subject – every bit as much a man as the physician-investigator. Fidelity is between man and man in these procedures. Consent expresses or establishes this relationship, and the requirement of consent sustains it. Fidelity is the bond between consenting man and consenting man in these procedures. The principle of an informed consent is the cardinal *canon of loyalty* joining men together in medical practice and investi-

6. *The Patient as Person*, New Haven, Conn.: Yale University Press, 1970, pp 2-11.
7. Report of the Judicial Council, E G Shelley, MD, Chairman, and approved by the House of Delegates of the American Medical Association, June 1968.

gation. In this requirement, faithfulness among men – the faithfulness that is normative for all the covenants or moral bonds of life with life – gains specification for the primary relations peculiar to medical practice.

Consent as a canon of loyalty can best be exhibited by a paraphrase of Reinhold Niebuhr's celebrated defence of democracy on both positive and negative grounds: 'Man's capacity for justice makes democracy possible; man's propensity to injustice makes democracy necessary.'[8] Man's capacity to become joint adventurers in a common cause makes the consensual relation possible; man's propensity to overreach his joint adventurer even in a good cause makes consent necessary. In medical experimentation the common cause of the consensual relation is the advancement of medicine and benefit to others. In therapy and in diagnostic or therapeutic investigations, the common cause is some benefit to the patient himself; but this is still a joint venture in which patient and physician can say and ideally should both say, 'I cure.'. . .

The foregoing paragraphs describe the basis of the requirement that experimentation involving human subjects should be undertaken only when an informed consent has been secured. There are enormous problems, of course, in knowing how to subsume cases under this moral regulation expressive of respect for the man who is the subject in medical investigations no less than in applying this same moral regulation expressive of the meaning of medical care. What is and what is not a mature and informed consent is a preciously subtle thing to determine. Then there are questions about how to apply this rule arising from those sorts of medical research in which the patient's knowing enough to give an informed consent may alter the findings sought; and there is debate about whether the use of prisoners or medical students in medical experimentation, or paying the participants, would not put them under too much duress for them to be said to consent freely even if fully informed. Despite these ambiguities, however, to obtain an understanding consent is a minimum obligation of a common enterprise and in a practice in which men are committed to men in definable respects. The *faithfulness*-claims which every man, simply by being a man, places upon the researcher are the morally relevant considerations. This is the ground of the consent-rule in medical practice, though obviously medical practice has also its consequence-features.

Indeed, precisely because there are unknown future benefits and precisely because the results of the experimentation may be believed to be so important as to be overriding, this rule governing medical experimentation upon human beings is needed to ensure that for the sake of those consequences no man shall be degraded and treated as a thing or as an animal in order that good may come of it. In this age of research medicine it is not only that medical benefits are attained by research but also that a man rises to the top in medicine by the success and significance of his research. The likelihood that a researcher would make a mistake in departing from a generally valuable rule of medical practice because he is biased toward the research benefits of permitting an 'exception' is exceedingly great. In such a seriously important moral matter, this should be enough to rebut a policy of being open to future possible exceptions to this canon of medical ethics. On grounds of the faithfulness-claims alone, we must surely say that future experience will provide no morally significant exception to the requirement of an informed consent – although doubtless we may learn a great deal more about the meaning of this particular canon of loyalty, and how to apply it in new situations with greater sensitivity and refinement – or we may learn more and more how to practice violations of it.

Doubtless medical men will always be learning more and more about the specific meaning which the requirement of an informed consent has in practice. Or they could learn more and more how to violate or avoid this requirement. But they are

---

8. *The Children of Light and the Children of Darkness*, New York, Scribner's, 1949, p.xi.

not likely to learn that it more and more does not govern the ethical practice of medicine. It is, of course, impossible to demonstrate that there could be *no* exceptions to this requirement. But with regard to unforeseeable future possibilities or apparently unique situations that medicine may face, there is this rule-assuring, principle-strengthening, and practice-upholding rule to be added to the requirement of an informed consent. In the grave moral matters of life and death, of maiming or curing, of the violation of persons or their bodily integrity, a physician or experimenter is more liable to make an error in moral judgment if he adopts a policy of holding himself open to the possibility that there may be significant, future permission to ignore the principle of the consent than he is if he holds this requirement of an informed consent always relevant and applicable. If so, he ought as a practical matter to regard the consent-principle as closed to further morally significant alteration or exception. In this way he braces himself to respect the personal subject while he treats him as patient or tries procedures on him as an experimental subject for the good of mankind.

The researcher knows that his judgment will generally be biased by the fact that he strongly desires one of the consequences (the rapid completion of his research for the good of mankind) which he could hope to attain by breaking or avoiding the requirement of an informed consent. This, too, should strengthen adherence in practice to the principle of consent. If every doer loves his deed more than it ought to be loved, so every researcher his research – and, of course, its promise of future benefits for mankind. The investigator should strive, as Aristotle suggested, to hit the mean of moral virtue or excellence by 'leaning against' the excess or the defect to which he knows himself, individually or professionally, and mankind generally in a scientific age, to be especially inclined. To assume otherwise would be to assume an equally serene rationality on the part of men in moral matters. It would be to assume that a man is as able to sustain good moral judgment and to make a proper choice with a strong interest in results obtainable by violating the requirement of an informed consent as he would be if he had no such interest.

Thus the principle of consent is a canon of loyalty expressive of the faithfulness-claims of persons in medical care and investigation. Let us grant that we cannot theoretically rule out the possibility that there can be exceptions to this requirement in the future. This, at least, is conceivable in extreme examples. It is not logically impossible. Still this is a rule of the highest human loyalty that ought not in practice to be held open to significant future revision. To say this concerning the there and then of some future moral judgment would mean here and now to weaken the protection of coadventurers from violation and self-violation in the common cause of medical care and the advancement of medical science. The material and spiritual pressures upon investigators in this age of research medicine, the collective bias in the direction of successful research, the propensities of the scientific mind toward the consequences alone are all good reasons – even if they are not all good moral reasons – for strengthening the requirement of an informed consent. This helps to protect coadventurers in the cause of medicine from harm and from harmfulness. This is the edification to be found in the thought that man's propensity to overreach a joint adventurer even in a good cause makes consent necessary.

This negative aspect of the ethics of medical research is essential even if only because the constraints of the consent-requirement serve constantly to drive our minds back to the positive meaning or warrant for this principle in the man who is the patient and the man who performs these procedures. An informed consent alone exhibits and establishes medical practice and investigation as a voluntary association of free men in a common cause. The negative constraint of the consent-requirement serves its positive meaning. It directs our attention always upon the man who is the patient in all medical procedures and a partner in all investigations, and away from that celebrated 'non-patient,' the future of medical science. Thus consent lies at the heart of medical care as a joint adventure between patient and doctor. It lies at the heart of man's continuing search for cures to all man's diseases as a great human adventure that is carried forward jointly by the investigator and his subjects. Stripped of the requirement of a reasonably free and an adequately informed consent, experimentation and medicine itself would speedily become inhumane.

No one today would propose to eliminate the consent-requirement directly, but this can be done more subtly, or by indirection. Even while retaining it, the consent-requirement can be effectively annulled, or transformed into a disappearing, powerless guideline, simply by writing into it a 'quantity-of-benefits-to-come' -exception clause. Thus we could make ourselves ready to override or avoid the consent-requirement in view of future good to be achieved. To do this is to make ourselves conditionally willing to use a subject in medical investigations as a mere means.

Extract 2: George J. Annas: Baby Fae[9]

Was Baby Fae a brave medical pioneer whose parents chose the only possible way to save her life, or was she a pathetic sacrificial victim whose dying was exploited and prolonged on the altar of scientific progress? To answer this question we need to examine the historical context of this experiment, together with the actions and expressed motives of the parents and physicians.

In an exclusive interview in *American Medical News* ten days after he had transplanted the heart of a baboon into Baby Fae, Dr Leonard Bailey described Dr James D Hardy as 'my silent champion.' Speaking of Dr Hardy's transplant of a chimpanzee heart into a human being in 1964, he said, 'He's an idol of mine because he followed through and did what he should have done . . . he took a gamble to try to save a human life.'[10]

Dr Hardy of the University of Mississppi, did the world's first lung transplant on a poor, uneducated, dying patient who was serving a life sentence for murder. John Richard Russell survived the transplant for seventeen days, and died as a result of kidney problems that were expected to kill him in any event. Less than seven months later, in January 1964, Dr. Hardy performed the world's first heart transplant on a human being, using the heart of a chimpanzee. The recipient of the chimpanzee heart, Boyd Rush, did not consent to the procedure. Like Mr Russell, he was dying and poor. Although not a prisoner, he was particularly vulnerable because he was a deaf-mute. He was brought to the hospital unconscious and never regained consciousness. A search for relatives turned up only a stepsister who was persuaded to sign a consent form authorizing 'the insertion of a suitable heart transplant' if this should prove necessary. The form made no mention of a primate heart; in later written reports Dr Hardy contended that he had discussed the procedure in detail with *relatives*, although there was only one. Mr Rush survived two hours with the chimpanzee heart.

Dr Hardy's justifications for using the chimpanzee heart were the difficulty of obtaining a human heart and the apparent success of Dr Keith Reemtsma in transplanting chimpanzee kidneys into Jefferson Davis at New Orleans Charity Hospital. Mr Davis was a forty-three-year-old poor black man who was dying of glomerulonephritis. Davis describes his consent in this transcript of a conversation with his doctors after the operation:

---

9. 'Baby Fae: The "Anything Goes" School of Human Experimentation', *The Hastings Center Report*, February 1985, pp.15-17.
10. This and later quotes by Dr Bailey appear in Dennis L Breo, 'Interview with "Baby Fae's" Surgeon: Therapeutic Intent was Top-most,' *American Medical News*, Nov.16, 1984, p.1.

*You told me that's one chance out of a thousand. I said I didn't have no choice
. . . You told me it gonna be animal kidneys. Well, I ain't had no choice.*[11]

The operation took place on November 5, 1963; the patient was doing well on
November 18 when he was visited by Dr Hardy. On December 18 he was released
to spend Christmas at home. Two days later he was back in hospital, and on
January 6, 1964, he died.

Whatever else one wants to say about these transplants, it is doubtful that
anyone would seriously attempt to justify either the consent procedures or the
patient selection procedures. Both experiments took advantage of poor, illiterate,
and dying patients for their own research ends. Both seem to have violated the
major precepts of the Nuremberg Code regarding voluntary, competent, informed,
and understanding consent; sufficient prior animal experimentation; and an *a priori*
reason to expect death as a result of the experiment.

The parallels are striking. Like Russell, Rush, and Davis, Baby Fae was
terminally ill; her dying status was used against her as the primary justification for
the experiment. We recognize that children, prisoners, and mental patients are at
special risk for exploitation, but the terminally ill are even more so, with their dying
status itself used as an excuse to justify otherwise unjustifiable research. Like
these previous subjects, Baby Fae was also impoverished; subjects in xenograft
experiments have 'traditionally' been drawn from this population. Finally, as a
newborn, she was even more vulnerable to exploitation. . . .

The Reasonableness of the Experiment

While different accounts have been given, it seems fair to accept the formulation
by immunologist Dr Sandra Nehlsen-Cannarella: 'Our hypothesis is that a new-
born can, with a combination of its under-developed immune system and the aid
of the anti-suppressive drug, cyclosporine, accept the heart of a baboon if we can
find one with tissue of high enough comparability.'[12] Questions that need answers
are: Is there sufficient animal evidence to support this 'underdeveloped immune
system' hypothesis as reasonable in the human? Does the evidence give any
reason to anticipate benefit to the infant? And is there any justification for
experimenting on infants before we experiment on adults who can consent for
themselves? The answer to all three questions seems to be no.

Only two new relevant scientific developments have occurred since the 1963-
64 experiments of Reemtsma and Hardy: better tissue-matching procedures and
cyclosporine. Both of these, however, are equally applicable to adults. Only the
'underdeveloped immune system' theory, which posits that transplants are more likely
to succeed if done in infants with underdeveloped immune systems, is applicable to
newborns, and this could be tested equally well with a human heart. Without this type
of prior work we are engaged, as one of my physician colleagues puts it, in 'dog
lab' experiments, using children as means to test a hypothesis rather than as
ends in themselves. Without adult testing, there could be no reasonable anticipation
of benefit for this child; the best that could be hoped for is that the parents would
bury a very young child instead of an infant. There should be no more xenografts
on children until they have proven successful on adults.

The Consent Process

On day ten after Baby Fae's transplant Dr Bailey said:

In the best scenario, Baby Fae will celebrate her 21st birthday without the
need for further surgery. That possibility exists.

---

11. Material about Dr Hardy is drawn from Jurgen Thorwald, *The Patients*, New York, Harcourt
Brace Jovanovich, 1972.
12. See note 11 above.

This was, in fact, never a realistic or reasonable expectation, and raises serious questions both about Dr Bailey's ability to separate science from emotion, and what exactly he led the parents of Baby Fae to expect. He seemed more honest when he described the experiment as a 'tremendous victory' after Baby Fae's death. But this could only mean that the experiment itself was the primary end, and that therapy was never a realistic goal.

As of this writing the Baby Fae consent form remains a Loma Linda Top Secret Document. But the process is much more important than the form, and it has been described by the principals. Minimally, there should have been an independent patient selection committee to screen candidates to ensure that the parents could not easily be taken advantage of, could supply the child with sufficient stable support to make long-term survival possible, were aware of all reasonable alternatives in a timely manner, and were not financially constrained in their decision making.

Baby Fae's parents had a two-and-a-half-year-old son, had been living together for about four years, had never married, and had been separated for the few months prior to Baby Fae's birth. Her mother is a high school dropout who was forced to depend on Aid to Families with Dependent Children at the time of the birth of Baby Fae. Baby Fae's father had three children by a previous marriage and describes himself as a middle-aged adolescent. He was not present at the birth of Baby Fae and did not learn about it until three days later. Both felt guilty about Baby Fae's condition, and wanted to do 'anything' that might 'save her life.'

Dr Bailey describes the crux of the consent process as a conversation with the parents from about midnight until 7 a.m. on October 20. In Dr Bailey's words:

> Apparently, the parents had spent three or four hours in debate at home [before admitting the baby] and now, from midnight until well into the next morning, I spent hours talking to them very candidly and very frankly. While Baby Fae was resting in bed, I showed them a film and I gave them a slide show, explaining our research and our belief why a baboon heart might work.

This account, given slightly more than two weeks after the transplant, is in error. Apparently Dr Bailey is following Dr Hardy's precedent of exaggerating the number of 'relatives' involved in the consent process. What really happened is recounted by the couple in their exclusive interview in *People* magazine. Present at the midnight explanation were not 'the parents,' but the mother, the grandmother, and a male friend of the mother who was staying at her home at the time of Baby Fae's birth. Baby Fae's father was *not* in attendance, although he says, 'I would have been there at the meeting with Dr Bailey if I'd known it was going to turn into a seven-hour discussion." Nonetheless, even though he missed the explanations about what was going to happen to his daughter,' when it came time to sign the agreements, I was up there."[13]

It is unclear that either of the parents ever read or understood the consent forms, but it is evident that the father was not involved in any meaningful way in the consent process.

Lessons of the Case

This inadequately reviewed, inappropriately consented to, premature experiment on an impoverished, terminally ill new-born was unjustified. It differs from the xenograft experiments of the early 1960s only in the fact that there was prior review of the proposal by the IRB (Institutional Review Board). But this distinction did not make a difference for Baby Fae. She remained unprotected from ruthless experimentation in which her only role was that of victim.

---

13. Information and quotes concerning Baby Fae's parents are taken from Eleanor Hoover, 'Baby Fae: A Child Loved and Lost,' *People*, Dec. 3, 1984, pp.49-63. The second part of the interview appeared in the Dec.10 issue.

Dr David B Hinshaw, the Loma Linda spokesman, understood part of the problem. In responding to news reports that the hospital might have taken advantage of a couple in 'different circumstances to wrest things from them in terms of experimental procedures,' he said that if this was true, 'The whole basis of medicine in Western civilization is challenged and attacked at its very roots.'[14] This is an overstatement. Culpability lies at Loma Linda.

Some will find this indictment too harsh. It may be (although none of us can yet know) that the IRB followed the NIH rules on research involving children to the letter, and that the experiments *could* be fit into the federal regulations by claiming that Baby Fae's terminally ill status was justification for an attempt to save her life. But if the federal regulations cannot prevent this type of gross exploitation of the terminally ill, they must be revised. We may need a 'national review board' to deal with such complex matters as artificial hearts, xenographs, genetic engineering, and new reproductive technologies. That Loma Linda might be able to legally 'get away with' what they have done demonstrates the need for reform and reassertion of the principles of the Nuremberg Code.

As philosopher Alasdair MacIntyre told a recent graduating class of Boston University School of Medicine, there are two ways to be a bad doctor. One is to break the rules; the other is to follow all the rules to the letter and to assume that by so doing you are being 'good.' The same can be said of IRBs. We owe experimental subjects more that the cold 'letter of the law.'

The *Loma Linda University Observer*, the campus newspaper, ran two headline stories on November 13, 1984, two days before Baby Fae's death. The first headline read '. . . And the beat goes on for Baby Fae'; the second, which covered an unconnected social event, could have more aptly captioned the Baby Fae story: 'Almost Anything Goes' comes to Loma Linda.'

Extract 3: Willard Gaylin: Harvesting the Dead[15]

In the ensuing discussion, the word *cadaver* will retain its usual meaning, as opposed to the new cadaver, which will be referred to as a *neomort*. The 'ward' or 'hospital' in which it is maintained will be called a *bioemporium* (purists may prefer *bioemporion*).

Whatever is possible with the old embalmed cadaver is extended to an incredible degree with the neomort. What follows, therefore, is not a definite list but merely the briefest of suggestions as to the spectrum of possibilities.

TRAINING: Uneasy medical students could practice routine physical examinations – auscultation, percussion of the chest, examination of the retina, rectal and vaginal examinations, et cetera – indeed, everything except neurological examinations, since the neomort by definition has no functioning central nervous system.

Both the student and his patient could be spared the pain, fumbling, and embarrassment of the 'first time.'

Interns also could practice standard and more difficult diagnostic procedures, from spinal taps to pneumoencephalography and the making of arteriograms, and residents could practice almost all of their surgical skills – in other words, most of the procedures that are now normally taught with the indigent in wards of major city hospitals could be taught with neomorts. Further, students could practice more exotic procedures often not available in a typical residency – eye operations, skin grafts, plastic facial surgery, amputation of useless limbs, coronary surgery, etc.; they could also practice the actual removal of organs, whether they be kidneys, testicles, or what have you, for delivery to the transplant teams.

14. *New York Times*, Nov. 15, 1984, pp. 27.
15. *Harpers Magazine*, September 1974, pp.23-30

TESTING: The neomort could be used for much of the testing of drugs and surgical procedures that we now normally perform on prisoners, mentally retarded children, and volunteers. The efficacy of a drug as well as its toxicity could be determined beyond limits we might not have dared approach when we were concerned about permanent damage to the testing vehicle, a living person. For example, operations for increased vascularization of the heart could be tested to determine whether they truly do reduce the incidence of future heart attack before we perform them on patients. Experimental procedures that proved useless or harmless could be avoided; those that succeed could be available years before they might otherwise have been. Similarly, we could avoid the massive delays that keep some drugs from the marketplace while the dying clamor for them.

Neomorts would give us access to other forms of testing that are inconceivable with the living human being. We might test diagnostic instruments such as sophisticated electrocardiography by selectively damaging various parts of the heart to see how or whether the instrument could detect the damage.

EXPERIMENTATION: Every new medical procedure demands a leap of faith. It is often referred to as an 'act of courage,' which seems to me an inappropriate terminology now that organized medicine rarely uses itself as the experimental body. Whenever a surgeon attempts a procedure for the first time, he is at best generalizing from experimentation with lower animals. Now we can protect the patient from too large a leap by using the neomort as an experimental bridge.

Obvious forms of experimentation would be cures for illnesses which would first be induced in the neomort. We could test antidotes by injecting poison, induce cancer or virus infections to validate and compare developing therapies. . .

BANKING: While certain essential blood antigens are readily storable (e.g. red cells can now be preserved in a frozen state), others are not, and there is increasing need for potential means of storage. Research on storage of platelets to be used in transfusion requires human recipients, and the data are only slowly and tediously gathered at great expense. Use of neomorts would permit intensive testing of platelet survival and probably would lead to a rapid development of a better storage technique. The same would be true for white cells.

As has been suggested, there is great wastage in the present system of using kidney donors from cadavers. Major organs are difficult to store. A population of neomorts maintained with body parts computerized and catalogued for compatibility would yield a much more efficient system. Just as we now have blood banks, we could have banks for all the major organs that may someday be transplantable – lungs, kidney, heart, ovaries. Beyond the obvious storage uses of the neomort, there are others not previously thought of because there was no adequate storage facility. Dr Marc Lappé of the Hastings Center has suggested that a neomort whose own immunity system had first been severely repressed might be an ideal 'culture' for growing and storing our lymphoid components. When we are threatened by malignancy or viral disease, we can go to the 'bank' and withdraw our stored white cells to help defend us.

HARVESTING: Obviously, a sizeable population of neomorts will provide a steady supply of blood, since they can be drained periodically. When we consider the cost-benefit analysis of this system, we would have to evaluate it in the same way as the lumber industry evaluates sawdust – a product which in itself is not commercially feasible but which supplies a profitable dividend as a waste from a more useful harvest.

The blood would be a simultaneous source of platelets, leukocytes, and red cells. By attaching a neomort to an IBM cell separator, we could isolate cell types at relatively low cost. The neomort could also be tested for the presence of hepatitis in a way that would be impossible with commercial donors. Hepatitis as a transfusion scourge would be virtually eliminated.

Beyond the blood are rarer harvests. Neomorts offer a great potential source of bone marrow for transplant procedures, and I am assured that a bioemporium of modest size could be assembled to fit most transplantation antigen requirements. And skin would, of course, be harvested – similarly, bone, corneas, cartilage, and so on.

MANUFACTURING: In addition to supplying components of the human body, some of which will be continually regenerated, the neomort can also serve as a manufacturing unit. Hormones are one obvious product, but there are others. By the injection of toxins, we have a source of antitoxin that does not have the complication of coming from another animal form. Antibodies for most of the major diseases can be manufactured merely by injecting the neomort with the viral or bacterial offenders.

Perhaps the most encouraging extension of the manufacturing process emerges from the new cancer research, in which immunology is coming to the fore. With certain blood cancers, great hope attaches to the use of antibodies. To take just one example, it is conceivable that leukemia could be generated in individual neomorts – not just to provide for *in vivo* (so to speak) testing of anti-leukemic modes of therapy but also to generate antibody immunity responses which could then be used in the living...

If seen only as the harvesting of products, the entire feasibility of such research would depend on intelligent cost-benefit analysis. Although certain products would not warrant the expense of maintaining a community of neomorts, the enormous expense of other products, such as red cells with unusual antigens, would certainly warrant it. Then, of course, the equation is shifted. As soon as one economically sound reason is found for the maintenance of the community, all of the other ingredients become gratuitous by-products, a familiar problem in manufacturing. There is no current research to indicate the maintenance cost of a bioemporium or even the potential duration of an average neomort. Since we do not at this point encourage sustaining life in the brain-dead, we do not know the limits to which it could be extended. This is the kind of technology, however, in which we have previously been quite successful.

Meantime, a further refinement of death might be proposed. At present we use total brain function to define brain death. The source of electro-encephalogram activity is not known and cannot be used to distinguish between the activity of higher and lower brain centers. If, however, we are prepared to separate the concept of 'aliveness' from 'personhood' in the adult, as we have in the fetus, a good argument can be made that death should be defined not as cessation of total brain function but merely as cessation of cortical function. New tests may soon determine when cortical function is dead. With this proposed extension, one could then maintain neomorts without even the complication and expense of respirators. The entire population of decorticates residing in chronic hospitals and now classified among the incurably ill could be redefined as dead...

And yet, after all the benefits are outlined, with the lifesaving potential clear, the humanitarian purposes obvious, the technology ready, the motives pure, and the material costs justified – how are we to reconcile our emotions? Where in this debit-credit ledger of limbs and livers and kidneys and costs are we to weigh and enter the repugnance generated by the entire philanthropic endeavor?

Cost-benefit analysis is always least satisfactory when the costs must be measured in one realm and the benefits in another. The analysis is particularly skewed when the benefits are specific, material, apparent, and immediate, and the price to be paid is general, spiritual, abstract, and of the future. It is that which induces people to abandon freedom for security, pride for comfort, dignity for dollars. . . .

The argument can be made on both sides. The unquestionable benefits to be gained are the promise of cures for leukemia and other diseases, the reduction of suffering, and the maintenance of life. The proponents of this view will be mobilized with a force that may seem irresistible.

They will interpret our revulsion at the thought of a bioemporium as a bias of our education and experience, just as earlier societies were probably revolted by the startling notion of abdominal surgery, which we now take for granted. The proponents will argue that the revulsion, not the technology, is inappropriate.

Still there will be those, like May, who will defend that revulsion as a quintessentially human factor whose removal would diminish us all, and extract a price we cannot anticipate in ways yet unknown and times not yet determined. May feels that there is 'a tinge of the inhuman in the humanitarianism of those who believe that the perception of social need easily overrides all other considerations and reduces the acts of implementation to the everyday, routine, and casual.'[16]

This is the kind of weighing of values for which the computer offers little help. Is the revulsion to the new technology simply the fear and horror of the ignorant in the face of the new, or is it one of those components of humanness that barely sustain us at the limited level of civility and decency that now exists, and whose removal is one more step in erasing the distinction between man and the lesser creatures – beyond that, the distinction between man and matter?

Sustaining life is an urgent argument for any measure, but not if that measure destroys those very qualities that make life worth sustaining.

Questions: Human Experimentation

1. If experimenting on X will produce greater happiness than unhappiness for society, then it is permitted to perform the experiment. Would it make any difference to your decision if X was a) a terminal cancer patient; b) a convicted murderer; c) a brain-dead baby; d) a cadaver; e) a monkey?

2. 'Since a foetus cannot consent to an experiment being performed upon it, all foetal experimentation is morally improper.' Discuss.

3. Was Baby Fae patient or victim?

4. Construct a deontological argument against the Baby Fae experiment?

5. Construct a deontological argument against harvesting the dead.

6. Two groups of soldier may benefit from penicillin: 1) those suffering from venereal disease; and 2) those suffering from infected wounds. Should the first group be given priority on moral grounds, or the second because they can be restored to active duty more quickly?

7. 'A debt can be met by selling off my property, be it my house, my kidney or my foetus.' Discuss.

16. William May, 'Attitudes Toward the Newly Dead', *The Hastings Center Studies*, I , No.1, 1973.

8. A woman has a right to be free of an unwanted foetus; she does not have a right to decide what shall we done with it after its abortion.' Discuss.

9. 'Unless expressly forbidden by the descendent or next of kin, the law should presume permission for the post-mortem removal of organs.' Discuss.

10. 'Without experimenting on those who have Alzheimer's, no cure for the disease will be forthcoming.' Discuss in relation to the issue of consent.

ANIMAL EXPERIMENTATION

As we saw in a previous chapter, the right to life is invariably held to be a right of human beings and not of everything living.[17] If this were not assumed, weeding the garden or killing cattle would be morally equivalent to, say, infanticide. In other words, we take for granted that human life is above all other forms of life and that the life of a man, being of greater value than that of any other animal, deserves special protection. We have seen already how deep-seated this view is in our discussions of abortion and euthanasia. While we do not object to killing animals in testing foodstuffs or cosmetics, the termination of a pregnancy is surrounded by a host of moral and legal difficulties; and while it took Karen Quinlan's father many court appearances to get his daughter taken off a respirator (perhaps the most famous case of passive euthanasia) we know that there would be no such judicial qualms about slaughtering a number of monkeys to investigate drug addiction. Non-human life is thus considered inferior to human life and this allows us to use animals as we think fit, even to the point of killing them. In recent years, however, this position has been vigorously denied by a number of philosophers, who, because they do not see any morally relevant difference between human and animal life, see no reason why the life of a man should be accorded special protection. This in turn has led some activists to conduct a campaign of violence against butchers' shops, furriers, factory farms, and scientific establishments. For these people, the same arguments that forbid research on humans or eating infants forbid this being done to non-humans. Bombing the home of a vivisectionist is none the less illegal but it is not, therefore, ethically wrong: all that one is doing is intimidating a murderer.

The ethical problem that concerns us here is highlighted by Tom Regan in our first extract. There seems, he argues, considerable moral confusion in the favouritism we extend to ourselves and not to animals. The Baby Fae experiment is a case in point. We assume that a premature child has a right to life which takes precedence over any rights that another animal might have. But the animal that gave his life for Baby Fae was a 'somebody' and had a name – Goobers. Arguing from the premise that all primates have equal moral value, and quite apart from the question of whether the experiment produced any benefits, Regan condemns the operation because Goobers did not exist as Fae's resource.

This point is developed by the philosopher Peter Singer. For Singer the crucial question in this debate is: 'Is it ever right to treat one kind of thing in

---

17. See above, pp. 30-31

the way that we would not treat another kind?' His answer is that, if one entity shares an equal capacity with another to be harmed or benefited – particularly in the capacity to experience pleasure or pain – then, whatever other differences may exist between them, this equality requires us to treat them equally. This explains why we do not teach dogs to read just because we teach children to or extend to giraffes the right to vote or to stones the more general right of freedom from having pain inflicted on them: they do not share with humans an equal capacity to benefit or derive pleasure or pain from these things. On the other hand, if we denied other human beings these rights, simply because they were black and not white, we would be accused of racial discrimination, of denying them things from which they could benefit purely on the grounds of racial origin. But what, asks Singer, if the comparison is between a monkey and a severely retarded infant? Drawing the line here is not so easy since the capacities of the monkey – his ability to act, to solve problems, to communicate, not to mention his capacity to feel pleasure and pain – will almost certainly equal and probably surpass those of the child. Does this mean we would select the child rather than the monkey for our experiments? We would not.

Despite its evident superiority in capacity, then, the monkey would still be chosen *because it is not biologically a member of our own species*. Goobers would always be selected before human beings, no matter what their medical condition, even before, for example, anencephalic babies lacking normal brain function. But to do this is morally unacceptable since it flouts the rights of the baboon to equal treatment. The animal, indeed, is the victim of another form of discrimination – not racism but **speciesism** – which is widely practised by all those who, while protecting the right to life of senile humans or human foetuses or brain-damaged humans, see no reason to stop the wholesale and wanton slaughter of non-human animals.

Singer's argument is opposed by Carl Cohen in our final extract. Cohen trumpets the fact that he is a speciesist, and condemns animal liberation not only as intellectually confused but as morally atrocious. Animals, he argues, have no inalienable right to life because having this right – indeed, having *any* right – depends on the capacity to make free moral decisions, which no animal possesses. Because, therefore, human beings have this capacity, they alone have membership of a 'moral community' from which animals are necessarily excluded. Membership, however, imposes upon them certain obligations towards each other, such as the duty of saving lives, which could not be upheld if animals were not used in scientific experiments. Cohen believes that the utilitarian argument here is a powerful one, and that to refrain from using animals in biomedical research is morally wrong. Human beings must secure for each other the greatest possible balance of pleasure over pain, and therefore must seek the elimination of disease. In calculating how this can be achieved, the advantages of using animals far outweigh the disadvantages of not using them. To maximise the protection of human subjects, the use of animal subjects should therefore be encouraged rather than discouraged. To extend the use of animals is part of the moral obligation that human beings have to one another.

Extract 4: Tom Regan: The Other Victim[18]

Like most people, my heart broke when Baby Fae died. It was no good my telling myself that thousands of babies die every day. Baby Fae was special. A member of our extended family, she was a child of the nation. When she died, we all grieved.

Others on this occasion will be drawn to debate the ethics of her treatment. I shall not here defend, only voice, my conviction that she was not treated fairly, that her interests were not uppermost in the aspirations of her principal caregivers. On this occasion I am pulled in another direction. For, unlike some people, my heart broke twice during Baby Fae's public struggle. There were two victims, in my view, not just one, though, like the proverbial black cat in the dark room, the other victim was easy to overlook.

In grieving Baby Fae's death, we were on familiar ground. She was *somebody*, a distinct individual with an unknown but partly imaginable future. If we allowed ourselves, we could share her first taste of ice cream, feel the butterflies in her stomach before the third grade play, endure her braces. When we consider the other victim, the baboon, the landscape changes. That lifeless corpse, the still beating heart wrenched from the uncomprehending body: for some people that death marks the end, not of somebody, but of some *thing*. A member of some species. A model. A tool. A token of a type. After all, there were no braces, there was no junior prom, in that brute creature's future.

Lack of empathy for the baboon is not easily improved upon. Even to note its absence or, more boldly, to suggest the appropriateness of our grieving over 'its' death will meet with stiff incredulity in some quarters. When the choice is between a baby and a baboon, can there be any question? Really?

However natural it may seem to answer 'no,' I think we must answer 'yes.' It is true that Goobers (though seldom used, this was the baboon's name) had a quite different potential, a quite different future form of life than Baby Fae. But no one, surely, will seriously question whether the duration and quality of his life mattered to that animal. Surely no one will seriously suggest that it was a matter of indifference to Goobers whether he kept his heart or had it transferred to another. Are we not yet ready to see that creatures such as baboons not only are alive, they have a life to live?

The weary charges of 'anthropomorphism' will fill the air. Baboons feel pain, it may be allowed. But their sentience exhausts their psychology. A twinge of discomfort here, maybe a warm stroke of pleasure there; that about does it.

This sparse view of baboon psychology will not stand up under the weight of our best thinking, neither philosophical nor scientific. Baboons not only feel pain, they *prefer* to avoid it, *remember* what it is like, *intentionally* seek to avoid it, *fear* its source. To describe and explain baboon behaviour in such mentalistic terms is intelligible, confirmable, and defensible. As Darwin saw, and as we should see, the psychology of such creatures differs from ours in degree, not in kind. Like us, Goobers was *somebody*, a distinct individual. He was the experiencing subject of a life, a life whose quality and duration mattered to him, independently of his utility to us.

Suppose this is true. Where does it take us morally? Everything depends on how firm the moral status of experiencing subjects-of-a-life is believed to be. You are such a subject, and so am I. Morally, I do not believe that you exist *for me*, as my resource, to be used by me to forward my own or, for that matter, someone else's interests. And, of course, I do not believe that I exist as your resource either. Just as I would violate your right to be treated with respect if I forced my will on you in the name of promoting my own or anyone else's welfare, so you would

18. *The Hastings Center Report*, February 1985, pp.9-10

do the same to me if you treated me similarly. This sort of strict equality between us, viewed as experiencing subjects-of-a-life, is, I believe, the fundamental precept in terms of which the morality of all our interactions ultimately must be gauged.

I would appeal to this precept to defend my opposition to using a healthy Baby Fae's heart to save the life of a sick Goobers. She did not exist as his resource. But I would insist upon equal treatment for Goobers. He did not exist as her resource either. Those people who seized his heart, even if they were motivated by their concern for Baby Fae, grievously violated Goober's right to be treated with respect. That he could do nothing to protest, and that many of us failed to recognize the transplant for the injustice that it was, does not diminish the wrong, a wrong settled before Baby Fae's sad death. Fundamental moral wrongs are not alterable by future results. Or past intentions.

What, then, can we do when, as is certain, we face other Baby Faes whose life hangs by a thread? Morally and medically, we must do everything we may, balancing, as best we can, the vital interests present in health care contexts such as these against those we find in others. With limited resources, we cannot, alas, do everything it would be good to do. What we must not do, either now or in the future, is violate the rights of some in order to benefit others. Our gains must be well, not ill, gotten. One measure of our medical progress will be the number of Baby Faes we are able to keep alive. But our resolve not to kill future Goobers will be one measure of our moral growth.

Extract 5: Peter Singer: All Animals are Equal[19]

If a being suffers, there can be no moral justification for refusing to take that suffering into consideration. No matter what the nature of the being, the principle of equality requires that its suffering be counted equally with the like suffering – in so far as rough comparisons can be made – of any other being. If a being is not capable of suffering, or of experiencing enjoyment or happiness, there is nothing to be taken into account. This is why the limit of sentience (using the term as a convenient, if not strictly accurate shorthand for the capacity to suffer or experience enjoyment or happiness) is the only defensible boundary of concern for the interests of others. To mark this boundary by some characteristic like intelligence or rationality would be to mark it in an arbitrary way. Why not choose some other characteristic, like skin colour?

The racist violates the principle of equality by giving greater weight to the interests of members of his own race, when there is a clash between their interests and the interests of those of another race. Similarly the speciesist allows the interests of his own species to override the greater interests of members of other species. The pattern is the same in each case. Most human beings are speciesists. I shall now very briefly describe some of the practices that show this.

For the great majority of human beings, especially in urban, industrialized societies, the most direct form of contact with members of other species is at mealtimes: we eat them. In doing so we treat them purely as means to our ends. We regard their life and well-being as subordinate to our taste for a particular kind of dish. I say 'taste' deliberately – this is purely a matter of pleasing our palate. There can be no defense of eating flesh in terms of satisfying nutritional needs, since it has been established beyond doubt that we could satisfy our need for protein and other essential nutrients far more efficiently with a diet that replaced animal flesh by soy beans, or products derived from soy beans, and other high protein vegetable products.

It is not merely the act of killing that indicates what we are ready to do to other

19. Peter Singer, 'All Animals are Equal', *Philosophic Exchange*, 2 (1974). Abridged reprint in *Applied Ethics*, ed. Singer, Oxford, Oxford University Press, 1986, pp. 222-25

species in order to gratify our tastes. The suffering we inflict on the animals while they are alive is perhaps an even clearer indication of our speciesism than the fact that we are prepared to kill them. In order to have meat on the table at a price that people can afford, our society tolerates methods of meat production that confine sentient animals in cramped, unsuitable conditions for the entire duration of their lives. Animals are treated like machines that convert fodder into flesh, and any innovation that results in a higher 'conversion ratio' is liable to be adopted. . . .

Since, as I have said, none of these practices cater to anything more than our pleasure of taste, our practice of rearing and killing other animals to eat them is a clear instance of the sacrifice of the most important interests of other beings in order to satisfy trivial interests of our own. To avoid speciesism we must stop this practice, and each of us has a moral obligation to cease supporting this practice. Our custom is all the support that the meat industry needs. The decision to cease giving it that support may be difficult, but it is no more difficult than it would have been for a white Southerner to go against the traditions of his society and free his slaves; if we do not change our dietary habits, how can we censure those slaveholders who would not change their own way of living?

The same form of discrimination may be observed in the widespread practice of experimenting on other species in order to see if certain substances are safe for human beings, or to test some psychological theory about the effect of severe punishment on learning, or to try out various new compounds just in case something turns up. . . .

In the past, argument about vivisection has often missed the point, because it has been put in absolutist terms: would the abolitionist be prepared to let thousands die if they could be saved by experimenting on a single animal? The way to reply to this purely hypothetical question is to pose another: would the experimenter be prepared to perform his experiment on an orphaned human infant, if that were the only way to save many lives? (I say 'orphan' to avoid the complication of parental feelings, although in doing so I am being overfair to the experimenter, since the non-human subjects of experiments are not orphans). If the experimenter is not prepared to use an orphaned human infant, then his readiness to use non-humans is simple discrimination, since adult apes, cats, mice and other mammals are more aware of what is happening to them, more self-directing and, so far as we can tell, at least as sensitive to pain, as any human infant. There seems to be no relevant characteristic that human infants possess that adult mammals do not have to the same or a higher degree. (Someone might try to argue that what makes it wrong to experiment on a human infant is that the infant will, in time and if left alone, develop into more than the non-human, but one would then, to be consistent, have to oppose abortion, since the foetus has the same potential as the infant – indeed, even contraception and abstinence might be wrong on this ground, since the egg and sperm, considered jointly, also have the same potential. In any case, this argument still gives us no reason for selecting a non-human, rather than a human with severe and irreversible brain damage, as the subject for our experiments.)

The experimenter, then, shows a bias in favour of his own species whenever he carries out an experiment on a non-human for a purpose that he would not think justified him in using a human being at an equal or lower level of sentience, awareness, or ability to be self-directing. No one familiar with the kind of results yielded by most experiments on animals can have the slightest doubts that if this bias were eliminated, the number of experiments performed would be a minute fraction of the number performed today. . . .

Extract 6: Carl Cohen: The Case for the Use of Animals in Biomedical Research[20]

Using animals as research subjects in medical investigations is widely condemned on two grounds: first, because it wrongly violates the *rights* of animals, and second, because it wrongly imposes on sentient creatures much avoidable *suffering*. Neither of these arguments is sound. The first relies on a mistaken understanding of rights; the second relies on a mistaken calculation of consequences. Both deserve definitive dismissal.

WHY ANIMALS HAVE NO RIGHTS

A right, properly understood, is a claim, or potential claim, that one party may exercise against another. The target against whom such a claim may be registered can be a single person, a group, a community, or (perhaps) all humankind. The contents of rights claims also varies greatly: repayment of loans, nondiscrimination by employers, noninterference by the state, and so on. To comprehend any genuine right fully, therefore, we must know *who* holds the right, *against whom* it is held, and *to what* it is a right.

Alternative sources of rights add complexity. Some rights are grounded in constitution and law (e.g. the right of an accused to trial by jury); some rights are moral but give no legal claims (e.g. my right to your keeping the promise you gave me); and some rights (e.g. against theft or assault) are rooted both in morals and in law.

The differing targets, contents, and sources of rights, and their inevitable conflict, together weave a tangled web. Notwithstanding all such complications, this much is clear about rights in general: they are in every case claims, or potential claims, within a community of moral agents. Rights arise, and can be intelligibly defended, only among beings who actually do, or can, make moral claims against one another. Whatever else rights may be, therefore, they are necessarily human; their possessors are persons, human beings. . . .

Animals (that is, nonhuman animals, the ordinary sense of that word) lack this capacity for free moral judgment. They are not beings of a kind capable of exercising or responding to moral claims. Animals therefore have no rights, and they can have none. This is the core of the argument about the alleged rights of animals. The holders of rights must have the capacity to comprehend rules of duty, governing all including themselves. In applying such rules, the holders of rights must recognize possible conflicts between what is in their own interest and what is just. Only in a community of beings capable of self-restricting moral judgments can the concept of a right be correctly invoked.

Humans have such moral capacities. They are in this sense self-legislative, are members of communities governed by moral rules, and do possess rights. Animals do not have such moral capacities. They are not morally self-legislative, cannot possibly be members of a truly moral community, and therefore cannot possess rights. In conducting research on animal subjects, therefore, we do not violate their rights, because they have none to violate. . . .

A common objection, which deserves a response, may be paraphrased as follows:

> If having rights requires being able to make moral claims, to grasp and apply moral laws, then many humans – the brain-damaged, the comatose, the senile – who plainly lack those capacities must be without rights. But

20. *The New England Journal of Medicine*, vol.315, No. 14 (October, 1986) pp.865-869

that is absurd. This proves [the critic concludes] that rights do not depend
on the presence of moral capacities.

This objection fails; it mistakenly treats an essential feature of humanity as though
it were a screen for sorting humans. The capacity for moral judgment that distinguishes humans from animals is not a test to be administered to human beings
one by one. Persons who are unable, because of some disability, to perform the
full moral functions natural to human beings are certainly not for that reason ejected
from the moral community. The issue is one of kind. Humans are of such a kind
that they may be the subject of experiments only with their voluntary consent. The
choices they make freely must be respected. Animals are of such a kind that it is
impossible for them, in principle, to give or withhold voluntary consent or to make a
moral choice. What humans retain when disabled, animals have never had.

A second objection, also often made, may be paraphrased as follows:
   Capacities will not succeed in distinguishing humans from the other animals. Animals also reason; animals also communicate with one another;
   animals also care passionately for their young; animals also exhibit desires and preferences. Features of moral relevance – rationality, interde-
   pendence, and love – are not exhibited uniquely by human beings. Therefore [this critic concludes], there can be no solid moral distinction between
   humans and other animals.

This criticism misses the central point. It is not the ability to communicate or to
reason, or dependence on one another, or care for the young, or the exhibition of
preference, or any such behavior that marks the critical divide. Analogies between
human families and those of monkeys, or between human communities and those
of wolves, and the like, are entirely beside the point. Patterns of conduct are not at
issue. Animals do indeed exhibit remarkable behavior at times. Conditioning, fear,
instinct, and intelligence all contribute to species survival. Membership in a
community of moral agents nevertheless remains impossible for them. Actors
subject to moral judgment must be capable of grasping the generality of an ethical
premise in a practical syllogism. Humans act immorally often enough, but only
they – never wolves or monkeys – can discern, by applying some moral rule to the
facts of a case, that a given act ought or ought not to be performed. The moral
restraints imposed by humans on themselves are thus highly abstract and are
often in conflict with the self-interest of the agent. Communal behavior among
animals, even when most intelligent and most endearing, does not approach
autonomous morality in this fundamental sense.

   Genuinely moral acts have an internal as well as an external dimension. Thus,
in law, an act can be criminal only when the guilty deed, the actus reus, is done
with a guilty mind, mens rea. No animal can ever commit a crime; bringing animals to criminal trial is the mark of primitive ignorance. The claims of moral right
are similarly inapplicable to them. Does a lion have a right to eat a baby zebra?
Does a baby zebra have a right not to be eaten? Such questions, mistakenly
invoking the concept of right where it does not belong, does not make good sense.
Those who condemn biomedical research because it violates 'animal rights' commit
the same blunder.

IN DEFENSE OF 'SPECIESISM'
Abandoning reliance on animal rights, some critics resort instead to animal sentience
– their feelings of pain and distress. We ought to desist from the imposition of pain
insofar as we can. Since all or nearly all experimentation on animals does impose

pain and could be readily forgone, say these critics, it should be stopped. The ends sought may be worthy, but those ends do not justify imposing agonies on humans, and by animals the agonies are felt no less. The laboratory use of animals (these critics conclude) must therefore be ended – or at least very sharply curtailed.

Argument of this variety is essentially utilitarian, often expressly so; it is based on the calculation of the net product, in pains and pleasures, resulting from experiments on animals. Jeremy Bentham, comparing horses and dogs with other sentient creatures, is thus commonly quoted: 'The question is not, Can they reason? nor Can they talk? but, Can they suffer?'

Animals certainly can suffer and surely ought not to be made to suffer needlessly. But in inferring, from these uncontroversial premises, that biomedical research causing animal distress is largely (or wholly) wrong, the critic commits two serious errors.

The first error is the assumption, often explicitly defended, that all sentient animals have equal moral standing. Between a dog and a human being, according to this view, there is no moral difference; hence the pains suffered by dogs must be weighed no differently from the pains suffered by humans. To deny such equality, according to this critic, is to give unjust preference to one species over another; it is 'speciesism.' The most influential statement of this moral equality of species was made by Peter Singer:

> The racist violates the principle of equality by giving greater weight to the interests of members of his own race when there is a clash between their interests and the interests of those of another race. The sexist violates the principle of equality by favoring the interests of his own sex. Similarly the speciesist allows the interests of his own species to override the greater interests of members of other species. The pattern is identical in each case.[21]

This argument is worse than unsound; it is atrocious. It draws an offensive moral conclusion from a deliberately devised verbal parallelism that is utterly specious. Racism has no rational ground whatever. Differing degrees of respect or concern for humans for no other reason than that they are members of different races is an injustice totally without foundation in the nature of the races themselves. Racists, even if acting on the basis of mistaken factual beliefs, do grave moral wrong precisely because there is not morally relevant distinction among the races. The supposition of such differences has led to outright horror. The same is true of the sexes, neither sex being entitled by right to greater respect or concern than the other. No dispute here.

Between species of animate life, however – between (for example) humans on the one hand and cats or rats on the other – the morally relevant differences are enormous, and almost universally appreciated. Humans engage in moral reflection; humans are morally autonomous; humans are members of moral communities, recognizing just claims against their own interest. Human beings do have rights; theirs is a moral status very different from that of cats or rats.

I am a speciesist. Speciesism is not merely plausible; it is essential for right conduct, because those who will not make the morally relevant distinctions among species are almost certain, in consequence, to misapprehend their true obligations. The analogy between speciesism and racism is insidious. Every sensitive moral judgment requires that the differing natures of the beings to whom obligations are owed be considered. If all forms of animate life – or vertebrate animal life? – must be treated equally, and if therefore in evaluating a research program the pains of a rodent count equally with the pains of a human, we are forced to conclude (1) that neither humans nor rodents possess rights, or (2) that rodents possess all the rights that humans possess. Both alternatives are absurd. Yet one or the other

21. See above, p. 91

must be swallowed if the moral equality of all species is to be defended.

Humans owe to other humans a degree of moral regard that cannot be owed to animals. Some humans take on the obligation to support and heal others, both humans and animals, as a principal duty in their lives; the fulfilment of that duty may require the sacrifice of many animals. If biomedical investigators abandon the effective pursuit of their professional objectives because they are convinced that they may not do to animals what the service of humans requires, they will fail, objectively, to do their duty. Refusing to recognize the moral differences among species is a sure path to calamity. . . .

Those who claim to base their objection to the use of animals in biomedical research on their reckoning of the net pleasures and pains produced make a second error, equally grave. Even if it were true – as it is surely not – that the pains of all animate beings must be counted equally, a cogent utilitarian calculation requires that we weigh all the consequences of the use, and of the nonuse, of animals in laboratory research. Critics relying (however mistakenly) on animal rights may claim to ignore the beneficial results of such research, rights being trump cards to which interest and advantage must give way. But an argument that is explicitly framed in terms of interest and benefit for all over the long run must attend also to the disadvantageous consequences of not using animals in re-search, and to all the achievements attained and attainable only through their use. The sum of the benefits of their use is utterly beyond quantification. The elimination of horrible disease, the increase of longevity, the avoidance of great pain, the saving of lives, and the improvement of the quality of lives (for humans and for animals) achieved through research using animals is so incalculably great that the argument of these critics, systematically pursued, establishes not their conclusion but its reverse: to refrain from using animals in biomedical research is, on utilitarian grounds, morally wrong.

When balancing the pleasures and pains resulting from the use of animals in research, we must not fail to place on the scales the terrible pains that would have resulted, would be suffered now, and would long continue had animals not been used. Every disease eliminated, every vaccine developed, every method of pain relief devised, every surgical procedure invented, every prosthetic device implanted – indeed, virtually every modern medical therapy is due, in part or in whole, to experimentation using animals. Nor may we ignore, in the balancing process, the predictable gains in human (and animal) well-being that are probably achievable in the future but that will not be achieved if the decision is made now to desist from such research or to curtail it.

Medical investigators are seldom insensitive to the distress their work may cause animal subjects. Opponents of research using animals are frequently in-sensitive to the cruelty of the results of the restrictions they would impose. Untold numbers of human beings – real persons, although not now identifiable – would suffer grievously as the consequence of this well-meaning but shortsighted ten-derness. If the morally relevant differences between humans and animals are borne in mind, and if all relevant considerations are weighed, the calculation of long-term consequences must give overwhelming support for biomedical research using animals. . . .

Questions: Animal Experimentation

1. In the light of Regan's and Cohen's arguments, analyse the claim that Goobers had no rights.

2. What is it that makes human superior to animals and animals superior to humans? Do these differences justify speciesism?

3. What is your moral attitude to the transplantation of animal organs into the human body?

4. 'But so far as animals are concerned, we have no direct duties. Animals . . . are there merely as a means to an end. That end is man. . . . Our duties towards animals are merely indirect duties towards humanity" (Kant). Comment on this argument.

5. Are animal rights activists justified in conducting a campaign of violence against those who practise speciesism?

6. To what extent do advances in medical science justify animal experimentation?

7. Every new technique in medical science must be tested for safety. Should these tests be performed on animals rather than humans?

8. If animal liberation is a consistent and justified position, why is it that so few people are willing to adopt thoroughgoing vegetarianism is matters of food, clothing, and so on?

9. Consider the following statement: 'On an ethical scale, we will always place human beings ahead of subhumans, especially in a situation where people can be genuinely saved by animals. That is the story of mankind from the very beginning. Animals, for example, have always been used for food and clothing.'[22]

10. Is the comparison between speciesism and racism justified?

Bibliography

1) Human Experimentation

* denotes text extracted in main text

Alexander, Leo 'Medical Science under Dictatorship', *The New England Journal of Medicine*, 241, No.2, 14 July 1949, pp.39-47. A survey of the medical atrocities committed by the Nazis.

Annas, George 'Baby Fae: The "Anything Goes" School of Human Experimentation',* *Hastings Center Report*, 15 (1), February 1985, pp.15-17

– (edited with Michael Grodin). *The Nazi Doctors and the Nuremburg Code: Human Rights in Human Experimentation*, New York, Oxford University Press, 1992.

Gaylin, Willard 'Harvesting the Dead',* *Harpers Magazine*, September 1974, pp.23-30.

Jones, James *Bad Blood*, New York, Free Press, 1981. A detailed account of the Tuskegee Syphilis Study.

Kushner, Thomasine & Raymond Belotti. 'Baby Fae: A Beastly Business,' *Journal of Medical Ethics*, 11 (1985) pp.178-183.

22. 'Interview with Dr Jack Provonsha' (Director, Center for Christian Bioethics, Loma Linda Hospital), *U. S. News & World Report*, 12 November, 1984, p.59.

May, William 'Attitudes Toward the New Dead,' *The Hastings Centre Studies*, 1, No.1, 1973.

Lifton, Robert J. *The Nazi Doctors: Medical Killing and the Psychology of Genocide*, New York, Basic Books, 1986.

Pence, Gregory E *Classic Cases in Medical Ethics*, New York, McGraw-Hill, 1990. Ch.9 includes an excellent summary of the Tuskegee Syphilis Study.

Ramsey, Paul *The Patient as Person*,* New Haven & London, Yale University Press, 1970.

2) Animal Experimentation

Cohen, Carl 'The Case for the Use of Animals in Biomedical Research,'* *The New England Journal of Medicine*, vol. 315, No.14, October 1986, pp.865-870

Frey, R G *Rights, Killing and Suffering: Moral Vegetarianism and Applied Ethics*, Oxford: Basil Blackwell, 1983.

Godlovitch, R & S (ed. with J Harris), *Animals, Men and Morals*, London, Victor Gollancz, 1971.

Linzey, Andrew *Animal Rights*, London, SCM Press, 1976. An argument from the Christian perspective.

Magel, Charles *Keyguide to Information Sources in Animal Rights*, London, Mansell, 1989; and Macfarland, Jefferson, N.C., 1989. Extremely useful general bibliography.

Miller, H B (ed. with W H Williams). *Ethics and Animals*, Clifton, NJ: Humana Press, 1983.

Noske, Barbara *Humans and Other Animals*, London, PlutoPress,1989. Examination by an anthropologist of those animal activities previously thought to be exclusively human.

Regan, Tom *The Case for Animal Rights*, Berkeley, Calif., University of California Press, 1983.

– 'The Other Victim',* *Hastings Center Review*, 15 (1), February 1985, pp. 9-10.

Rollin, Bernard E *Animal Rights and Human Morality*, Buffalo, NY: Prometheus Books, 1981.

Ryder, Richard *Victims of Science*, London, Davis-Poynter, 1975; & London, National Anti-Vivisection Society, 1983.

Scruton, Roger *Animal Rights and Wrongs*, London, Demos, 1996. A spirited attack on Animal Liberation.

Singer, Peter 'All Animals are Equal',* *Philosophic Exchange*, 2, No 2, 1974. Abridged reprint in *Applied Ethics*, ed. Peter Singer, Oxford, Oxford University Press, 1986) pp 215-228;

– *Animal Liberation*, London, Jonathan Cape, 1975. The most influential contemporary discussion of the issue.

– *Practical Ethics*, Cambridge, Cambridge University Press, 1979. Excellent introduction, concentrating on contemporary issues, particularly animal rights, euthanasia and abortion.

– (ed. with T Regan) *Animal Rights and Human Obligations*, Englewood Cliffs, NJ: Prentice-Hall, 1976)

– (ed.) *In Defence of Animals*, Oxford, Basil Blackwell, 1985.

Chapter Six
The Ethical Theory of Immanuel Kant

Thus far we have looked at two normative theories of ethics: egoism and utilitarianism. They have had much in common. Each maintains that there is a highest good, something which is good in itself, and that this alone must be the goal of the moral life. This intrinsic good they call pleasure or happiness. Each further maintains that an action is right or wrong according to whether it produces this highest good. In other words, both utilitarianism and egoism are **teleological** in character because each judges the morality of an action in terms of its consequences or effects. Where they differ is in their view of whose happiness should be taken into account. For the egoist, priority is given to the happiness of the individual. For the utilitarian, it is given to the greater collective happiness of everyone.

Neither of these theories, however, has much in common with the position which is known as **deontological** ethics. This, we recall, denies that any action is right because of its consequences: it is right only because it conforms to certain independently valid principles or rules, rules like 'Never harm anyone' or 'Never break your promises.' These rules are not held, then, because they promote the good but because they are good, because they provide the standard of what is right and wrong. It is true that keeping these rules may sometimes have disastrous results, as we shall see presently; but that alone can never justify the breaking of them.

It is now time to look more closely at deontological ethics, and in particular at one major problem it has left unresolved. If I am being told that certain rules have independent moral worth – independent, that is, of their possible consequences – and that I should adhere to them, then how do I know that the moral rule I think I ought to obey has moral worth? How do I know that it is a rule that I, and everybody else, ought to obey? After all, if your view of the world is different from mine, it seems likely that your good rule will not necessarily be my good rule. So how do I establish what *the* good rule is, the rule which is good for all and which demands absolute obligation from everyone? What we want, then, is some method of assessing the moral worth of rules, so that we can say of them that these, and not those, are to hold for others as well as for myself. What we require is some sort of test which will enable us to pinpoint the laws to be obeyed. For this we must turn to the most influential of all theories of deontological ethics: **the theory of Immanuel Kant.**

Immanuel Kant (1724-1804) is generally regarded as one of the most influential thinkers of the Western philosophical tradition, being one of the last philosophers to construct a complete philosophical 'system', comprehensive in scope and covering most of the major issues of philosophy. This achievement is all the more remarkable because Kant, on the face of it, was a man of very limited experience. He spent his entire life in the provincial town of Königsberg in East Prussia, first as a student, than as a private tutor, and finally as Professor of Logic and Metaphysics. He never married, he never travelled, and his life followed a rigid routine which rarely altered. The German poet, Heinrich Heine, has given us an amusing description of the impression Kant made upon his neighbours:

> The life of Immanuel Kant is hard to describe; he has indeed neither life nor history in the proper sense of the words. He lived an abstract, mechanical, old-bachelor existence, in a quiet remote street in Königsberg, an old city at the north-eastern boundary of Germany. I do not believe that the great cathedral clock of that city accomplished its day's work in a less passionate and more regular way than its countryman, Immanuel Kant. Rising from bed, coffee-drinking, writing, lecturing, eating, walking, everything had its fixed time; and the neighbours knew that it must be exactly half-past four when they saw Professor Kant, in his grey coat, with his cane in his hand, step out of his house door, and move towards the little limetree avenue, which is named, after him, the Philosopher's Walk. Eight times he walked up and down that walk at every season of the year; and when the weather was bad, his servant, old Lampe, was seen anxiously following him with a large umbrella under his arm, like an image of Providence. Strange contrast between the outward life of the man and his world-destroying thought. Of a truth, if the citizens of Königsberg had had any inkling of the meaning of that thought, they would have shuddered before him as before an executioner. But the good people saw nothing in him but a professor of philosophy; and when he passed at the appointed hour, they gave him friendly greetings – and set their watches.[1]

Although Kant's philosophy defies easy classification, one aspect of his thought should be emphasised at the beginning of our discussion. This is the importance that Kant, in common with other philosophers of the Enlightenment, attaches to man's **ability to reason**. Two of his greatest works, the *Critique of Pure Reason* (1781) and the *Critique of Practical Reason* (1788) testify to his belief that it is man's rational faculty, his capacity to think objectively and apart from his own circumstances or preferences, that distinguishes him from all other creatures. A human being is essentially a rational being, and it is this that constitutes his intrinsic dignity. More than that, reason binds man to man. Since reason, Kant argues, is an innate intellectual power existing more or less equally in all men, it enables the individual to resolve his problems in a way more or less acceptable to everyone. For example, if one person, reasoning logically, concludes that a particular argument is self-contradictory, then another person, going through the same argument and also reasoning logically, will arrive at the same conclusion. *Here reason dictates that their answers are the same.* Now, significantly enough, Kant holds that this is also true when we apply our reason to moral problems. If, for instance, I conclude, using my reason, that a particular action is right, then this, says Kant, is the conclusion that would be reached by anyone in my position. What is right for me, using my reason, is right for everyone, using their reason.

We can now see the direction Kant takes in his search for the test that will

---

1. Quoted by E W F Tomlin, *The Western Philosophers,* London, Hutchinson & Co., 1968, p.202.

decide which moral laws should be unconditionally obeyed. *This test will be found in the operation of reason.* This is so because, if reason is universal, the moral commands generated by reason will be universal and applicable to all men. All that remains to be seen is how reason creates these rules and what these rules are. For this we must turn to Kant's famous little book, *Groundwork of the Metaphysic of Morals* (1783).

THE GOOD WILL

In the *Groundwork* Kant says that, if a moral law is to be unconditionally and universally binding, it must contain something that is unconditionally and universally *good*, something that is *good in itself*, and the *highest good*. But what can this good be? Kant reviews various possibilities. There are the 'talents of the mind', like intelligence and judgement; there are qualities of character, like courage, resolution and perseverance; there are the so-called 'gifts of fortune', like power, wealth and honour; and lastly, there is the utilitarian suggestion, happiness. However, Kant rejects all these for the same reason: all are capable of making a situation *morally worse*. For example, if a criminal is intelligent or powerful or rich, his crimes are generally more serious. Similarly, if a torturer gains pleasure from his deeds, or a murderer honour from his crime, we think his actions more reprehensible, not less. All these qualities, therefore, whatever their individual merits, can on occasion create something thoroughly bad; and for this reason alone they cannot be called intrinsically good or, what Kant terms, 'good without qualification'. For what is good without qualification must be incapable of reducing the moral worth of any situation. This being the case, what does Kant himself propose as the greatest good? He writes:

> 'It is impossible to conceive anything at all in the world, or even out of it, which can be taken as good without qualification, except a **good will**.[2]

Being a good man means, therefore, having a good will: without it, one cannot be good. But what exactly is a 'good will'? The first thing to note is that the good will 'is not good because of what it effects or accomplishes – because of its fitness for attaining some proposed end.'[3]

In other words, the goodness of a good will is not derived from the goodness of its *results* – a point which underlines the deontological character of Kant's thought. After all, a murderer, willing evil, may inadvertently do good; but this unexpected turn of events would not transform his original evil desires into good ones: they remain evil, even though the consequence is good. Moreover, says Kant, if the moral value of the good will were to depend on its effects, it could no longer be considered of unconditional value. For in that case we would have to judge it merely as a means to an end, as an *instrumental* good, as a good dependent on the achievement of a result: it would not however be the *intrinsic* good, the good 'without qualification'.

In determining the moral worth of an action, whether it is or is not gov-

2. *Groundwork of the Metaphysic of Morals*, translated, with analysis and notes, by H J Paton in *The Moral Law*, London, Hutchinson & Co., 1972, p.59.
3. *Ibid.*, p.60.

erned by a good will, the consequences of that action are therefore irrelevant. For Kant, it is not what an act accomplishes that is decisive, but the motive behind the act: *it is having the right intention that makes the good will good*. But what kind of intention might this be? Kant's famous reply is that a good will's only motive is *to act for the sake of duty*. In other words, a person is good when their only motive for doing something is that it is their duty to do it.

This is by no means easy to understand. In order to help us at this point, Kant introduces the following examples:

> It certainly accords with duty that a grocer should not overcharge his inex-
> perienced customer; and where there is much competition a sensible shop-
> keeper refrains from so doing and keeps to a fixed and general price for
> everybody so that a child can buy from him just as well as anyone else.
> Thus people are served honestly; but this is not nearly enough to justify us
> in believing that the shopkeeper has acted in this way from duty or from
> principles of fair dealing; his interest required him to do so. We cannot
> assume him to have in addition an immediate inclination towards his cus-
> tomers, leading him, as it were out of love, to give no man preference over
> another in the matter of price. Thus the action was done neither from duty
> nor from immediate inclination, but solely from purposes of self-interest.[1]

Kant is here telling us what doing one's duty does not involve: it does not involve serving one's own interests. This grocer is honest because being honest is good for business, not because he believes it is his duty to be honest. If he does not cheat his customers, his profits will increase. He does not there-fore do what he does because it is his duty to do it, but because it serves his own ends. This, then, is not the good will at work. Of course, it may be the case that this particular grocer is also *by inclination* honest and trustworthy; that acting in this way comes naturally to him, and that he derives pleasure from it. But even this, Kant adds, does not indicate the presence of a good will. No special merit can be attached to someone who does what is natural to them, even though what they do coincides with what their duty demands. An ulterior motive still exists – to do what they *enjoy* rather than what their duty prescribes – and the possibility always remains that, if they no longer enjoyed doing it, they would do otherwise: they will be honest as long as it pleases them to be so. Thus, Kant concludes, their will fails to be the good will, just as if they had acted from self-interest.

In describing the man of good will, Kant is therefore describing the kind of motive or intention a man must have for his actions to be good. This motive, to repeat, must be entirely free from the persons self-interest or calculation of what the consequences will be of his actions. Nor is it distinguished by certain kinds of pleasurable emotion – by feelings of kindliness, generosity or love – because these have to do with a person's inclinations and not with the selfless will to do one's duty, regardless of personal desires. By contrast, the man of good will acts solely in accordance with duty and for the sake of duty; and his only motive for doing what is right is his awareness that it is the right thing to do. He does what is right because it is right, and for no other reason.

4. *Ibid.*, p.63

Exercise 1

Which of the following duties would Kant eliminate as examples of the good will at work? Give reasons for your answers.

It is my duty . . .
a. to preserve my life, even though I find life unbearable
b. to commit suicide when I find life unbearable
c. to keep my promise, even though my friend will suffer as a result
d. to steal that bread because my children are starving
e. to punish my child
f. to take care of my old parents because they took care of me
g. to take care of my old parents, even though they didn't take care of me
h. to refuse my son the blood transfusions that will save his life
i. as a parent to send my son to a good school
j. as a doctor to cure this patient, even though it is Adolf Hitler
k. as a motorist to obey traffic lights
l. as a Nazi to kill Jews

THE CATEGORICAL IMPERATIVE

We have learned that, according to Kant, the morally good man is the man of good will, and that the man of good will is the man who does his duty. An action, therefore, only has moral worth if it is done from duty. We have also learnt what doing one's duty does *not* involve: it has nothing to do with obeying one's inclinations, serving one's own interests, and is not estimated in terms of consequences. So far so good. We can at least say that we know what doing one's duty isn't; but we have still to discover what it is. Kant has still to tell us where our duty lies.

However, we do already know two things about this, as yet unnamed, duty. The first is that, since Kant has rejected the idea that the moral worth of an action lies in its results – the teleological position – he must subscribe to the only other alternative – the deontological position – and say that the moral worth of an action lies in its obedience to a particular rule or principle regardless of inclinations, self-interest or consequences. Thus, whatever this principle or law is, it is in obeying it that we do our duty.

The second thing we know about this duty is that it must be of universal application, applicable to everyone irrespective of their situation. Accordingly, it must appeal to that aspect of man's nature which already binds man to man, namely, to his reason. This duty, in other words, must be of such a kind that to obey it is to exercise the rational faculty and not to obey it is to fall into irrational confusion. In obeying this law, then, the man of good will is exercising his reason in a moral matter, and what he does is what every reasonable man would do in similar circumstance. Conversely, making an irrational decision is contrary to acting in obedience to one's duty. For Kant, what is contradictory is immoral.

What, then, is this supreme principle of morality? What is this rule or law that the man of good will consciously or unconsciously recognises when he obeys his duty? Kant calls it the **categorical imperative**. An imperative tells me which of my possible actions would be good, and it does this in the form of a command, expressed by the words 'I ought'. Kant gives three versions of the categorical imperative, the first and most important of which runs as follows: 'I ought never to act except in such a way that I can also will that my maxim should become a universal law.'[5]

Let us first note that this imperative or command is categorical, not hypothetical. A **hypothetical imperative** tells us what actions would be good solely as a means to something else, for example, 'If I want to lose weight, I must eat less'. The point here is that the imperative (to eat less) is dependent on the desire to achieve a certain result (to lose weight); but if I do not want to lose weight, the command would lose its force. Eating less, therefore, is not considered good in itself but only as a means to an end: it is an instrumental good.

The categorical imperative, on the other hand, is obeyed precisely because what it commands is accepted as being good in itself, as being an intrinsic good. The action is undertaken because of the very nature of the action itself and not because it is the means of achieving something else. Nor is consideration given to the possible consequences of the action. 'If you want to be respected, tell the truth' is a hypothetical imperative. The categorical equivalent, however, would read simply 'Tell the truth'. It is a command that must be obeyed for its own sake and not for any ulterior motive. All moral commands, says Kant, are of this type. The categorical imperative is the *imperative of morality*.

However, the most important feature of the categorical imperative is its emphasis on **universalizability** – the willing 'that my maxim should become a universal law' – for it is this, Kant tells us, that provides us with the method of pinpointing those laws which have universal moral worth. In other words, the test we have been looking for, the test that will tell us what rules *all of us* should obey, is whether or not the rule in question can be universalised or, as Kant puts it in another formulation, whether I can will that it become a 'law of nature'. What I must discover is whether this rule can be consistently acted upon by all those in similar circumstances; and here it is the *consistency* of the rule that is decisive. For inconsistency, we remember, is the essence of immorality because it strikes at the very basis of our nature as rational human beings. Thus any rule that, when universalised, becomes contradictory must be dismissed as immoral. So, for example, the command 'Always accept help and never give it' lacks moral worth. It would, of course, be quite possible for *you* to obey it, but it would be quite impossible for everybody to obey it. It could not be universalised because, if everybody refused to help, there would be no help to receive. Thus this imperative, when extended to everybody, is contradictory and cannot therefore be accepted as a genuine moral command. Here the inability to universalise entails the lack of moral worth.

To clarify his argument at this stage, Kant gives the following four examples:

5. *Ibid.*, p.67. Kant's third formulation is very similar: 'So act that your will can regard itself at the same time as making universal law through its maxim' (p.96).

1. A man feels sick of life as the result of a series of misfortunes that have mounted to the point of despair, but he is still so far in possession of his reason as to ask himself whether taking his own life may not be contrary to his duty to himself. He now applies the test 'Can the maxim of my action really become a universal law of nature?' His maxim is 'From self-love I make it my principle to shorten my life if its continuance threatens more evil than it promises pleasure.' The only further question to ask is whether this principle of self-love can become a universal law of nature. It is then seen at once that a system of nature by whose law the very same feeling whose function is to stimulate the furtherance of life should actually destroy life would contradict itself and consequently could not subsist as a system of nature and is therefore entirely opposed to the supreme principle of all duty.

2. Another finds himself driven to borrowing money because of need. He well knows that he will not be able to pay it back; but he sees too that he will get no loan unless he gives a firm promise to pay it back within a fixed time. He is inclined to make such a promise; but he has still enough conscience to ask 'Is it not unlawful and contrary to duty to get out of difficulties in this way?' Supposing, however, he did resolve to do so, the maxim of his action would be: 'Whenever I believe myself short of money, I will borrow money and promise to pay it back, though I know that this will never be done.' Now this principle of self-love or personal advantage is perhaps quite compatible with my own entire future welfare; only there remains the question 'Is it right?' I therefore transform the demand of self-love into a universal law and frame my question thus: 'How would things stand if my maxim became a universal law?' I then see straight away that this maxim can never rank as a universal law of nature and be self-consistent, but must necessarily contradict itself. For the universality of a law that everyone believing himself to be in need can make any promise he pleases with the intention not to keep it would make promising, and the very purpose of promising, itself impossible, since no one would believe he was being promised anything, but would laugh at utterances of this kind as empty shams.

3. A third finds in himself a talent whose cultivation would make him a useful man for all sorts of purposes. But he sees himself in comfortable circumstances, and he prefers to give himself up to pleasure rather than to bother about increasing and improving his fortunate natural aptitudes. Yet he asks himself further 'Does my maxim of neglecting my natural gifts, besides agreeing in itself with my tendency to indulgence, agree also with what is called duty?' He then sees that a system of nature could indeed always subsist under such a universal law, although (like the South Sea Islanders) every man should let his talents rust and should be bent on devoting his life solely to idleness, indulgence, procreation, and, in a word, to enjoyment. Only he cannot possibly will that this should become a universal law of nature or should be implanted in us as such a law by a natural instinct. For as a rational being he necessarily wills that all his powers should be developed, since they serve him, and are given him, for all sorts of possible ends.

4. Yet a fourth is himself flourishing, but he sees others who have to struggle with great hardships (and whom he could easily help); and he thinks 'What does it matter to me? Let every one be as happy as Heaven wills or as he can make himself; I won't deprive him of anything; I won't even envy him; only I have no wish to contribute anything to his well-being or to his support in distress!' Now admittedly if such an attitude were a universal law of nature, mankind could get on perfectly well – better no doubt than if everybody prates about sympathy and goodwill, and even takes pains, on occasion, to practise them, but on the other hand cheats where he can, traffics in human rights, or violates them in other ways. But although it is possible that a universal law of nature could subsist in harmony with this maxim, yet it is impossible to will that such a principle should hold everywhere as a law of nature. For a will which decided in this way would be in conflict with itself, since many a situation might arise in which the man needed love and sympathy from others, and in which, by such a law of nature sprung from his own will, he would rob himself of all hope of the help he wants for himself.[6]

These examples tell us more about the inherent contradictory nature of all immoral actions. In the first two examples we find what Kant calls **contradictions in the law of nature**. These involve rules that cannot even be conceived as universal because they are straightforwardly self-contradictory. Such a rule would be 'Do this but don't'. There are, however, other rules, just as impossible, which do not appear so at first. Take Kant's example of keeping promises. It would be quite possible for you or I to adopt the rule, 'Only keep your promises when it is in your interest to do so'; but what would happen if this rule were universalised? A contradiction results. For if everyone could, when convenient, make a false promise, no one would trust the promises of others; and if this happened, the very practice of promise-keeping, which this rule presupposes, would be destroyed.

In examples 3 and 4, we find what Kant calls **contradictions in the will**. It is quite possible to have rules which, unlike those just mentioned, are not contradictory in themselves but which the person involved could not possibly wish to see universalised. This is because the resulting situation *must* be totally unacceptable to him. Thus people who have no concern for others cannot wish that everybody should act like them because the situation might arise when they also need help. Even selfish people, pursuing their own interests, could not possibly want to live in a world in which no one helps them because pursuing their own interests may require this help. Here, then, the contradiction lies in the universalisation of a rule that might later be used against them.

Exercise 2

Are the following imperatives universalizable? If they are not, is this because they are contradictions in the *law of nature* or in the *will*?

a. Come first in examinations
b. Never speak until you are spoken to.
c. Do not give money to the poor.

6. *Ibid.*, pp. 85-86.

d. Sell all you have and give to the poor.

e. Jump the queue.

f. Lie when it is convenient to do so.

g. Shoot first and argue later.

h. Be different: dye your hair blue.

i. Keep the population down: abstain from sexual relations.

j. Take what you want.

k. Be polite: let the other person enter first.

l. Defend yourself but never start the fight.

In concluding this account of Kant's moral theory, it is worth repeating that at its heart stands the belief that rational beings should always treat all other rational beings equally and in the same way that they would treat themselves. This view is best expressed in Kant's second formulation of the categorical imperative, which is one of the great humanistic doctrines of the Enlightenment: 'Act in such a way that you always treat humanity, whether in your own person or in the person of any other, never simply as a means, but always at the same time as an end.'[7] Because human beings are rational beings, they have an inherent value: they are ends in themselves, counting equally one with another. Their value does not therefore consist in how they can be used by others, as means to ends: their value is intrinsic, not instrumental. The principle of universalization underlines this view of the intrinsic worth of individual men and women. Suicide is wrong because it involves a person's use of himself or herself as a means to escape an intolerable situation. Similarly, making false promises is wrong because it involves making use of someone else as a means to greater gain. As with the first formulation of the categorical imperative, the second requires that no rule of conduct which is applicable universally to all rational beings can either sanction action favouring one over another or prescribe conduct by which one being treats another as a means to an end. To do so is to demean oneself and thereby humanity at large.

Exercise 3

Analyse the following as examples of universalization:

a. Being a diabetic I have to have an insulin injection every day. Since it is right for me to do this, it is right for everybody to do this. Therefore everybody should have an insulin injection every day.

b. If I prefer pork to lamb, everybody should prefer pork to lamb.

c. Jesus was wrong to say 'Love your enemies' because, if everyone loved their enemies, there would be no enemies left to love.

---

7. *Ibid.*, p.91.

Exercise 4

According to Kant, where would your duty lie in the following examples? Where do you think your duty lies?

a. In his book *Les Misérables*, Victor Hugo tells the story of an escaped convict, Jean Valjean, who, living under an assumed name, becomes a town's major benefactor, employer, and mayor. Later he discovers that an old tramp has been arrested as Jean Valjean and sentenced to the galleys. The real Valjean considers it his duty to reveal his true identity and so save the tramp from unjust punishment.

b. A plane crashes in the Andes. Many passengers survive. However, no rescue comes and their food rapidly runs out. In this extreme situation, facing death by starvation, they consider it their duty to eat the flesh of those who did not survive the crash.

c. Mr and Mrs Smith are Jehovah's Witnesses. Their son, David, is involved in a serious accident and requires immediate surgery. His parents are not against the operation but will not allow a blood transfusion. This, they say, is against their religious beliefs. The doctors reply that without the transfusion, David will die.

Exercise 5

According to Kant, suicide is wrong. As he argues:

> to use the power of a free will for its own destruction is self-contradictory. If freedom is the condition of life it cannot be employed to abolish life and so to destroy and abolish itself. To use life for its own destruction, to use life for producing lifelessness, is self-contradictory. These preliminary remarks are sufficient to show that man cannot rightly have any power of disposal in regard to himself and his life, but only in regard to his circumstances.[8]

This viewpoint is challenged by the Roman Stoic philosopher and poet, Lucius Annaeus Seneca (c. 4 BC – AD 65). How far do you agree or disagree with Seneca's alternative?

> Life has carried some men with the greatest rapidity to the harbour, the harbour they were bound to reach even if they tarried on the way, while others it has fretted and harassed. To such a life, as you are aware, one should not always cling. For mere living is not a good, but living well. Accordingly, the wise man will live as long as he ought, not as long as he can. He will mark in what place, with whom, and how he is to conduct his existence, and what he is about to do. He always reflects concerning the quality, and not the quantity, of his life. As soon as there are many events in his life that give him trouble and disturb his peace of mind, he sets himself free. And this privilege is his, not only when the crisis is upon him, but as

8. *Lectures on Ethics*, trans. Louis Infield, New York, Harper & Row, 1963, pp.147-148.

soon as Fortune seems to be playing him false; then he looks about carefully and sees whether he ought, or ought not, to end his life on that account. He holds that it makes no difference to him whether his taking-off be natural or self-inflicted, whether it comes later or earlier. He does not regard it with fear, as if it were a great loss; for no man can lose very much when but a driblet remains. It is not a question of dying earlier or later, but of dying well or ill. And dying well means escape from the danger of living ill.[9]

SOME CRITICISMS AND AMENDMENTS OF KANT

The power of Kant's argument is undeniable and its importance has increased rather than diminished with the years. Various features of his theory remain particularly attractive.

The first is that it takes account of *justice*. More specifically, it corrects the utilitarian presumption that the morality of an action derives from the benefit produced or from the number of those who obtain that benefit, a view which puts the innocent at risk. This Kant does not allow. Punishment can never be justified in terms of majority benefit but is dependent solely on the intrinsic rightness or wrongness of the action performed. Justice towards the individual is thus safeguarded by the universal, and impartial, character of the categorical imperative, which imposes duties upon us all, equally and alike. An action taken against the individual, if contrary to duty, is therefore wrong, no matter how many may think otherwise.

Kant reaches the same conclusion from a different direction, namely, in his account of man as a being of intrinsic worth. Here it is each man's dignity as a *rational creature*, as the highpoint of creation, that resists all use of him as a mere means to an end, as something to be exploited for the greater happiness of others. This point of view is well illustrated by a remark Kant made just before his death. Although very sick and weak, Kant nevertheless struggled to his feet when his doctor entered the room and refused to sit down until his visitor had taken a chair. 'The feeling for humanity', he explained, 'has not yet left me.' This gesture is made, in other words, not because his guest is a doctor but because he is a human being. Here good manners is an expression of the respect to be accorded each man or woman as a rational being. This 'feeling for humanity' dominates Kant's entire philosophy.

Kant is also to be applauded for the sharp distinction he makes between duty and inclination. It prevents individuals from assuming that what is good for them, what brings them pleasure or benefit, is morally good, something that will be good for everyone. All of us are prone to make unjustifiable exceptions in our moral judgements – exceptions notably in favour of ourselves and our friends and to the detriment of those we dislike – but after Kant this becomes less excusable and, as a matter of logic, less consistent with the moral life. People of good will obey a law which is the same for all, and only thus do they subordinate their own natural inclinations, however generous these may be, become less self-centred and more appreciative of the rights of others.

9. 'On Suicide', in *Epistula Morales*, Loeb edition, vol.2, trans. Richard M Gummere, London, William Heinemann, 1970, pp.57-59.

This indeed is the great strength of universalisability. For me to assert that you ought to do X in situation Y commits me, as a matter of moral necessity, to the general rule that everyone should do things like X in situations like Y. In this way I perceive that my duties to others are no different from my duties to myself and that my rights are identical to theirs. As has been pointed out many times before, this is Kant's equivalent of the Golden Rule of Christian ethics: 'Do unto others as you would have them do unto you.'

Yet many find fault with Kant's position, in particular with his claim that moral people are those who must conduct their lives solely in obedience to the rules generated by the categorical imperative. For if this is the case, they argue, then doing one's duty must also include obeying rules towards which we feel no moral obligation whatsoever, or obeying rules which allow for the very exceptions that Kant sought to eliminate in his distinction between duty and inclination. Consider the following maxims:

1. Whenever anybody buys a new book, the purchaser should write his or her name on the fly-leaf.
2. Whenever anyone is over six feet tall, bald, without his right ear and little finger of his left hand, and working in Manchester as a nuclear physicist, he may be excused paying income tax.

The important thing to notice about these maxims is that neither is self-contradictory and that both are universalizable according to Kant's criteria (Whenever anyone is X, they are to do Y.) Yet, in the first example, we have a rule which is neither good nor bad but morally neutral, and which few would hold to be obligatory; and, in the second, a rule so precisely defined that it benefits no one but a particular individual. This being so, it cannot be correct to say, as Kant does, that the moral person is one who acts in accordance with the categorical imperative. For while there are many actions which the process of universalization rightly condemns, it is also quite possible, by the same procedure, to arrive at rules that the majority of us would consider either preferential or without moral significance. What these examples tell us, then, is that the ability of a rule to be universalised does not of itself guarantee that the rule will be morally good or even moral at all.

How, therefore, is the person of good will to decide whether a proposed rule is a good one? In his discussion of the so-called **contradictions in the will**, Kant suggests a way out of this difficulty, and indeed offers us a kind of practical test. We can reject those rules which, if universalised, would produce a state of affairs utterly objectionable to all rational people. Thus no individuals can rationally will that the helpless should never be helped because, as rational beings, they necessarily desire their own happiness, and to achieve this they will sometimes require the help of others. They must reject what is contrary to the objectives that all rational people must have.

But this is not very helpful. What Kant appears to overlook is that, while all people may be rational, we do not all have the same temperaments or desires, and that consequently *we do not all find the same situations intolerable*. Who is to say, for instance, that sadists would not wish to see sadism universalised? They might well prefer to have sadism universally practised, with themselves as both practitioners and victims, rather than to have no such practices at all. Similarly, thieves might well prefer stealing universalised, believing that they still stand to gain financially, even though their own property is at greater risk. Or consider Kant's own example of 'Never help the helpless'. Now it may well be true that rational beings, neither liking nor wanting to see their interests frustrated, will dislike this rule applying to themselves; but that is very different from saying that they will consider the universalization of this rule morally unjustified, that they will think this rule immoral when it applies to everybody, including themselves. Again, this depends on the temperament of the person concerned. A ruthless landlord, evicting his tenants, may well concede that he would not like the same thing happening to him; but that doesn't mean that he considers their eviction wrong, or that he wouldn't consider his own eviction right, if he were in their place. Indeed one suspects that there are many people who think like this, who accept that, just as they neglect others, others may neglect them. This, after all, is the capitalistic doctrine of self-help, according to which the individual realises that life is cut-throat and competitive and accepts the chance of failure in the pursuit of success. But there is nothing *irrational* in this. What would be irrational is if such an individual positively wanted his interests neglected or liked it when they were. There is nothing irrational in *a man of this type* accepting that others may treat him as ruthlessly as he treats others.

An equally damaging criticism can be made of Kant's so-called **contradictions in nature**. Telling lies or breaking promises is always wrong, he says, because neither can be consistently universalised. If we attempted to do so, we should quickly find the very business of telling the truth and keeping promises collapsing. For this reason the prohibition against lying and breaking promises is absolute and as such applies to everyone without exception.

But again, the problem lies in Kant's exclusion of exceptions. Must telling the truth always be right, irrespective of the circumstances in which I find myself? Can there be no situations in which, say, telling a lie is morally justified? There are, of course, many people who would agree with Kant about the absoluteness of certain rules. Conscientious objectors, who refuse to fight whatever the circumstances because 'life is sacred', are adopting his position, as indeed are those who oppose capital punishment for the same reason. But many others would disagree and say that there are times when making an exception is morally permissible: that fighting Hitler was one such exception and that hanging terrorists is another. Indeed, if exceptions are always disallowed, it is quite easy to imagine situations in which either no decision is possible or in which the decision made is morally reprehensible.

Take, for example, a situation where our duties conflict. If it is always wrong to break a promise and always wrong to tell a lie, what happens when I have to tell a lie to keep a promise? Suppose I promise a friend that I will hide him from a murderer, and that the murderer later asks me where my friend is. How am I to reply? If I tell the truth, I break a promise; and if I keep the promise, I must tell a lie. It is a major weakness of Kant's theory that it provides no answer to this dilemma. Most of us, however, would resolve it quite easily: we would introduce an exception to the rule about truth-telling, which would avoid the evil consequences of our friend's death (e.g. 'tell the truth, except when it leads to the death of an innocent person'). Making exceptions of this kind also helps us to resolve another problem. What would happen if I had made no promise to hide my friend? In that case, there is no conflict of duty and I am duty bound to tell the murderer the truth. In other words, if I do not here make an exception, my duty obliges me to do something which, in all probability, I regard as morally reprehensible. Thus, in these examples, Kant's theory leads either to a kind of moral stalemate, in which no moral decision can be made, or to a situation in which I may well regard doing my duty as being equivalent to doing wrong.

THE THEORY OF W. D. ROSS

It is because of problems like these that an important amendment has been made to Kant's ethics by the modern philosopher W D Ross (1877-1971.) Kantian duties, Ross argues, should not be taken as absolute duties but as duties *that allow exceptions*. These duties Ross calls **prima facie duties** (prima facie meaning 'at first sight'). A prima facie duty is a non-absolute or conditional duty, a duty which can always be overridden by a more compelling duty. So 'Never take a human life' is a prima facie duty: it is not something I must always do but something I must do only when it is not outweighed by another and more compelling obligation or rule of prima facie duty (e.g. 'Never take a human life except in self-defence'). Such obligations arise from the situations in which I find myself, and may, says Ross, be classified into six groups, of which the first two are past-looking and the rest future-looking:

> **1.** *Duties of fidelity* in which I act in accordance with a former promise of mine; and duties of reparation in which I act to make amends for my previous wrongful act.
> **2.** *Duties of gratitude* in which I act to repay a debt (i.e. services done by other men to me).
> **3.** *Duties of justice* in which I act to obtain an equal distribution of pleasure and happiness.
> **4.** *Duties of beneficence* in which I act to better the lot of others in respect of virtue or of intelligence or of pleasure.
> **5.** *Duties of self-improvement* in which I act to improve myself in respect of virtue or of intelligence.
> **6.** *Duties of nonmalificence* in which I refrain from doing people harm.[10]

To see how this works, let us take the duty of gratitude. If I see my father and a famous doctor drowning, whom should I save? The utilitarian, we remember, will urge me to save the doctor because of the greater good accruing to mankind. Yet many of us would find this advice repugnant because we have a special duty of gratitude to our parents, who have cared for us and supported us,

10. W. D. Ross, *The Right and the Good*, Oxford, Oxford University Press, 1930, p. 21

which outweighs any duty I might have to a stranger, no matter how much happiness his life will bring to the greater number. This, then, says Ross, is an entirely personal duty owed to a particular person on the basis of who they are and what they have done for us: it is also entirely past-looking and not future-looking.

As we shall see in a moment. Ross's list, which he admits is incomplete, presents its own problems. More immediately, his theory has the great merit of extending the range of our duties beyond that prescribed by Kant. Indeed, once we realise what is required of a duty to be absolute and exceptionless, we soon see that few, if any, duties can be regarded in this way. Invariably, there is some situation in which an absolute Kantian duty can be overridden. Thus, it is not enough to say with Kant that, for a duty to be a moral duty, it must be capable of consistent universalization. For as Ross indicates, there is no such thing as a rule without possible exceptions. In making these exceptions much will depend on the circumstance in which my duty is done, on the probable consequences of doing my duty, and on the personal relation that may exist between myself and those to whom I believe a duty is owed.

Exercise 6

Apart from saying that the duty of nonmaleficence is in general more binding than the duty of beneficence, Ross does not place his prima facie duties in any order of importance. One order has been suggested by Richard Purtill.[11] Do you agree with his ranking? If not, how would you alter or add to it?

a. Not to harm others
b. To make reparations for harm done to us
c. To keep our commitments
d. To repay our benefactors
e. To treat people as well as they deserve to be treated
f. To do some good to some people, deserving or not
g. To improve ourselves in some ways

There are two outstanding objections to Ross's theory:

1. How do we know what a prima facie duty actually is?
2. How do we know which prima facie duty to obey when there is a conflict between them?

Ross's reply to both questions is the same. Both the utilitarian and Kantian theories make the mistake of assuming that an absolute criterion of what is right and wrong can be found, the one using the criterion of pleasure, the other of duty. Given the infinite variety and range of our pleasures and duties, not to mention the infinite range of their effects, it was inevitable, says Ross, that no such criterion, whether teleological or deontological, could be achieved.

---

11. *Thinking About Ethics*, Englewood Cliffs, NJ: Prentice-Hall, 1976, p. 44. *The Right and the Good*, Oxford, Oxford University Press, 1930, p.21.

This is not to say, however, that our ethical decisions are without cognitive value. We simply *know* that acts like fulfilling a promise, or effecting a just distribution of good, or promoting the good of others are prima facie right; and we know that they are simply by consulting our deepest moral convictions. That these things are right is 'self-evident' to us, not in the sense that we have always known that they are, nor in the sense that we can prove that they are, but in the sense that 'we have reached sufficient mental maturity' just to know that they are. They have become, like the axioms of geometry or arithmetic, instances of knowledge and part of the fundamental nature of the universe. Ross continues:

> It would be a mistake to found a natural science on 'what we really think', i.e. on what reasonably thoughtful and well-educated people think about the subjects of the science before they have studied them scientifically. For such opinions are interpretations, and often misinterpretations, of sense-experience; and the man of science must appeal from these to sense-experience itself, which furnishes his real data. In ethics no such appeal is possible. We have no more direct way of access to the facts about rightness and goodness and about what things are right or good, than by thinking about them; the moral convictions of thoughtful and well-educated people are the data of ethics just as sense-perceptions are the data of a natural science. Just as some of the latter have to be rejected as illusory, so have some of the former; but as the latter are rejected only when they are in conflict with other more accurate sense-perceptions, the former are rejected only when they are in conflict with other convictions which stand better the test of reflection. The existing body of moral convictions of the best people is the cumulative product of the moral reflection of many generations, which has developed an extremely delicate power of appreciation of moral distinctions; and this the theorist cannot afford to treat with anything other than the greatest respect. The verdicts of the moral consciousness of the best people are the foundation on which he must build; though he must first compare them with one another and eliminate any contradictions they may contain.[12]

Many find this answer unsatisfactory. What would happen, for example, if a person decided that returning services rendered was not a prima facie duty or that the duty of retribution (not included in Ross's list) was? Presumably Ross would then claim that this person did not possess 'sufficient mental maturity' to make a proper judgement or had somehow misread his own mind, in which case this person's inner moral convictions cannot be considered, as Ross supposes, knowledge of self-evident truths. What we require here, and what Ross does not give us, is some method for determining when a person is morally mature and when he has read his moral convictions correctly. Moreover, to rely upon the moral convictions of other people as the data of ethics, albeit those who are thoughtful and well-educated, is to assume that these are the 'best people' precisely because they know what a prima facie duty is: that indeed they possess what Ross denied they could possess, namely, a criterion for deciding between a right and wrong action.

---

12. *Op.cit.*, pp. 40-41.

Exercise 7

How do you think Kant and Ross would resolve the following dilemmas? How would you resolve them?

a. A friend of yours, who once saved your life, has committed murder and asks you to hide him. Should you?

b. You are a trade union leader involved in a lengthy strike. Many of your members are already impoverished. Are you justified in relieving their distress by accepting funds from a universally despised foreign power?

c. Your child will die unless he undergoes an expensive operation. You are a poor man. Would you be justified in obtaining this money illegally?

d. A wife suspects that her husband, with whom she has been happily married for many years, is a spy. He is due to retire in a year. Should she inform the authorities immediately?

e. Would you be justified in blackmailing a landlord into reducing his rents in a seriously deprived area?

f. Would you, as a doctor, consider it your duty to inform the parents of a fourteen-year-old girl that she is using contraceptives?

g. You have information about a Mafia shipment of heroin into this country. If the shipment is seized by police, the Mafia will know you were the informer and will seek to kill you. Should you tell the police?

h. Your cellmate, who is old and dying, helps you escape and tells you where a large amount of money is hidden. His only condition is that you promise to support his family. You agree, find the treasure, but then discover that the business your family depends on is going bankrupt. Should you invest your cellmate's money?

RULE-UTILITARIANISM

In as much as it contains both deontological and teleological elements, Ross's theory is a hybrid. He accepts with Kant that there are certain rules of duty that we are obliged to fulfil (notably the past-looking duties of fidelity and gratitude); and at the same time he accepts with the utilitarians that we are not obliged to obey these rules if the consequences of so doing should prove disastrous. The fact that we have made a promise is always a strong moral reason for keeping it; but this promise may not hold in all circumstances and may be outweighed by more urgent obligations (notably by the future-looking duties of beneficence, self-improvement and nonmalifecence.)

Ross's theory has much in common with a further amendment of Kantian ethics: **rule-utilitarianism.** This, the last theory of normative ethics we shall examine, is also a hybrid: it agrees with Ross about the centrality of rules and also accepts that sometimes the consequences of obeying them require the breaking of them; but these conclusions are reached for very different reasons. Rule-utilitarianism has no concept of prima facie duty, it denies that there are any past-looking duties, and, above all, it provides an absolute criterion of judgement for making moral decisions. Accordingly many believe it overcomes the objections levelled against Ross.

It will be remembered that, following Bentham, the ultimate criterion of ethical judgment is the *principle of utility*: an action is right if it brings pleasure (or prevents pain) and wrong if it brings pain (and prevents pleasure.) But the principle of utility, here applying to actions – hence the more specific description of Bentham's theory as 'act-utilitarianism' – can equally well apply to rules. All we have to do is evaluate the rule in terms of whether anyone obeying it will maximise overall happiness or unhappiness. What we have to do, in other words, is determine whether, *if everyone obeyed this rule*, it would promote the greatest good or not. If it does, then any action which conforms to that rule will be deemed right and any that does not will be deemed wrong.

For example, consider the question, 'Should I drive on the left or the right?' If the reply to this is, 'Well, it depends on my needs at the time: it might be on the left one day and on the right the next,' the results would be clearly disastrous for motorists and pedestrians alike. For this reason one consults the law of the land, knowing that in this instance safety is best served by everybody doing the same thing. In other words, the principle of utility here dictates that everyone should act, and always act, in accordance with a specific rule. This avoids the hazards of individual choice. If the law states 'Always drive on the right,' then the action of doing so is right because it conforms to the law.

In act-utilitarianism, therefore, right action is determined solely by that action's consequences. In rule-utilitarianism right action is determined not by the action's consequences but by the consequences of the rule under which that action is performed. More precisely, what distinguishes the two forms of utilitarianism is the extent to which rule-utilitarianism *incorporates Kant's notion of universalisability*: it is the consequences of a rule's universalization which determine whether it is a good or bad rule. Where rule-utilitarianism parts company from Kant is in evaluating the rule in terms of its consequences and in therefore retaining the principle of utility as the ultimate criterion of all moral decision.

We can make this distinction clearer with another example. Suppose a teacher sees an able and otherwise reliable student cheating in an examination. Nobody else has seen him cheating and the examination is crucial for the student's career and for his young family. What should the teacher do? As an act-utilitarian he could argue that, given the disastrous consequences for the student, he should turn a blind eye particularly since this action, being performed in secret, cannot set a bad example to others. The rule-utilitarian, however, would argue differently. While the teacher in this particular case may do more good for this particular student by saying nothing, and while it may be true that saying nothing can have no consequences for future cases because nobody will ever find out, it is still a bad thing to do because if everybody did this the whole business of taking examinations would be undermined. The fact indeed that it was done in secret – which for the act-utilitarian was an important consideration in limiting the possible evil consequences of his action – only makes it worse because nobody would then know who was keeping silent and nobody would then know whether the results of any examination were accurate. Here, then, it is the disastrous consequences of universalizability which decide the issue. The belief that the teacher did wrong comes not from our conviction that cheating doesn't produce happiness – in the case of the student it probably did – but from our conviction that even greater unhappiness would result if we universalised the rule under which the teacher operated. The teacher's action is condemned, therefore, not because of what he did, but because, to put the matter in Kantian terms, the maxim of his action – 'Allow cheating if it produces happiness' – would, if universalised, have evil results. Here again utility determines which rule applies.

Exercise 8

How would a rule-utilitarian deal with the following commands?

a. Since everybody smokes in the cinema anyway, ignore the signs telling you not to.

b. Always help your own children more than other people's.

c. Try to escape from prison if the law has convicted you of a crime you didn't commit.

d. Steal from the rich to give to the poor.

e. If you disapprove of the war, escape the draft.

f. Never give a student extra marks in public but in secret only.

g. Don't become a vegetarian: too many people eat meat for your action to make any difference.

h. Catholic priests don't marry, so neither should you.

i. If a tax includes payment for nuclear weapons, don't pay it.

Rule-utilitarians maintain that their position resolves two outstanding issues: the problem of conflicting duties, which faced both Kant and Ross, and the problem of justice, which faced the act-utilitarians.

The Problem of Conflicting Duties

Ross, like Kant before him, provides no criterion by which to decide which duty to obey when duties conflict; all he claims is that the person concerned, through a process of introspection, will somehow know which to choose. Rule-utilitarianism, however, does appeal to an absolute criterion – the principle of utility – and it does so in such a way that the specific circumstances in which the conflict occurs are taken into account. For instance, consider again the Kantian dilemma: If 'Never break a promise' and 'Never tell a lie' are both categorical imperatives, what do I tell the murderer who wants to kill the friend I have promised to protect? If I tell him where my friend is, I break a promise; if I keep the promise, I must tell a lie.[13] What rule-utilitarianism asks here is: Which rule will maximise happiness in this particular case? Clearly telling a lie. In other words, the imperative 'Never break a promise' is rejected following the application of the principle of utility to the specific circumstances in which I find myself.

This procedure has two important implications for rule-making. The first is that, in tying the rule to the situation, it inevitably makes the rule more complicated. We are no longer faced with the simplicity of Kantian absolutes like 'Never kill' – a command given irrespective of consequences – but with a whole host of separate commands which may deal with killing in self-defence, killing in war, killing as a legal deterrent, killing as an act of mercy, and so on. But any of these rules, although more complicated, is still better than the Kantian rule because they address themselves to the actual rather than the general case and because any possible conflict of duty can be resolved through the empirical test of utility. This test, rule-utilitarians insist, is entirely future-looking, and applies even to such duties as making restitution for harm done or the obligation of gratitude to our parents. Once again these are upheld not because, as Ross maintained, they involve special prima facie duties to special people but because a society in which these rules are generally held will be better – that is, will be capable of maximizing happiness more effectively – than one in which they are not. Their assessment remains teleological.

The second implication for rule-making is as follows. For Kant and Ross the obligation to obey certain rules stands irrespective of the conditions existing in any particular society: their universality requires obedience no matter what the time or place. In rule-utilitarianism, however, the principle of utility generates rules that may be applicable to one society but not to another. For example, a rule to preserve the water supply will be beneficial in the Sahara but not in Scotland. A rule requiring rigorous birth control will be applicable in China but not in a seriously depopulated area. Not all rules, however, are of this character. There will be some rules that are so basic to the welfare of any society and the preservation of its citizens – for example, the rules against wantonly killing people – that they have universal application. The point to remember, however, is that the fact that people and societies disagree in their ethical judgements does not upset the normative ethical principle espoused by

13 See above, p. 111

rule-utilitarianism. Despite the historical or cultural differences that may exist between societies, it is still the rules generated by the principle of utility which will determine whether an action is right or wrong in any given case.

The Problem of Justice

It will be remembered that one of the criticisms levelled against act-utilitarianism was that it does not adequately take account of justice, does not secure an *equal distribution* of happiness and need not, therefore, deal with the individual according to his or her deserts or merits. Thus a utilitarian judge would be justified in condemning an innocent man to death if he or she believed that a greater good would result, such as restoring law and order.[14] Can the same criticism be levelled against rule-utilitarianism?

Needless to say, rule-utilitarians argue that it cannot. In the example just given, the question to ask is: 'What would be the consequences of having a rule which sanctioned the punishment of the innocent?' The effects would clearly be disastrous. The institution of such a rule – the general acceptance that punishment could be administered without regard to desert – would destroy our trust in the law, which is necessary for the maintenance of society, and induce in us a constant fear of arrest. It is, therefore, because rule-utilitarianism integrates the Kantian principle of universalizability with the principle of utility that it can see that justice is done to the individual; that indeed it can safeguard the rights of the citizen under the law by maintaining that, if the action of condemning an innocent person is wrong for me to do, it is wrong for everybody to do.

But here we hit a snag. In the argument just presented, justice is taken to be a part of utility, one of those conditions that goes towards maximizing happiness. But is it an essential condition? It would appear not. The rule-utilitarian is saying that justice is assured *only as long as* the general practice of being just actually does maximise happiness; but this implies also that, if justice doesn't do this, it can be jettisoned in favour of something else, something perhaps that we would now regard as blatantly unjust, something that does not secure an equal distribution of justice. Rule-utilitarianism has already allowed that different rules will be appropriate for different societies. In that case, it could be argued that slavery is justified in a country facing economic ruin through a labour shortage. But do we really want to say that slavery is just? It may in this instance achieve a greater balance of happiness over unhappiness but the slave is still a slave and forced to be so: he has become a slave not as a punishment for things he did but for the benefits he will bring to others (and in which he may not share.) A rule, therefore, that maximises happiness may yet be unjust in the way it distributes happiness. Thus, although rule-utilitarianism can accommodate justice in a way that act-utilitarianism cannot, it still provides no guarantee that it will. The principle of utility is, accordingly, double-edged – it may justify either justice or injustice; and, since everything depends on the situation at hand, there is no guarantee that utility will not be best served by injustice.

14. See above, p. 72

It is because of this objection that a final amendment is made to rule-utilitarianism, sometimes known as **extended rule-utilitarianism**. This involves making the principle of justice – or, more precisely, the principle of just distribution – not subordinate to but equal to the principle of utility. Justice is now no longer derivative but fundamental, an essential condition of moral action. Actions are, therefore, *deemed right or wrong according to the rules generated by the twin principles of utility and justice.* The principle of utility is upheld because the teleological (and utilitarian) proposition that people do have a moral obligation to secure a balance of happiness over unhappiness is accepted: but how this balance will be distributed can only be decided by the principle of justice. This principle is upheld, therefore, because the deontological (and Kantian) proposition that people have an intrinsic right to equal treatment is also accepted. This is not to say, however, that these two principles must always operate conjointly. Each can generate separate obligations. Thus, for example, we derive the obligation not to do injury primarily from the principle of utility, and the obligation to secure equality before the law primarily from the principle of justice; other obligations, like telling the truth or helping the underprivileged, may be properly construed from either. But however we may apportion rule to principle, it is on the basis of these two principles that rules can be constructed which will lead to a state in which a maximum balance of good over evil is as equally and extensively distributed as possible.

Those who adopt this amended form of rule-utilitarianism concede that sometimes the principles of utility and justice will conflict. It is, they say, difficult to accept that a small injustice can never win a greater justice or that unequal treatment can never produce a greater good. Is killing *never* right or truth-telling *never* wrong? The problem of conflict therefore remains; but if it does perhaps it should now be seen as an irreducible tension in the act of moral decision. All we can reasonably hope for is that, when these conflicts occur, the decisions we make will increase the sum total of human happiness while yet safeguarding the individual's right to be treated 'always as an end and never as a means only'.

Questions: The Theories of Kant and Ross

1. How does Kant base his ethics on the concept of reason?

2. How does the categorical imperative help decide between right and wrong action? Give examples when you think it does not help.

3. 'Don't do unto others as you would have them do unto you: their tastes may be different!' (George Bernard Shaw). Discuss.

4. Is George, who resisted the temptation to kill you, morally superior to Jack, who never thought of killing you at all? In what way does this question pose a problem for Kant's distinction between duty and inclination? How do you think Kant would resolve it?

5. Kant tells us to treat individuals 'always as an end and never as a means only.' Give examples in modern society of people being used as mere 'means.' What alternative treatments would you propose?

6. What problem is Ross's notion of prima facie duty trying to solve? Does it succeed?

7. Do you agree with Ross that we have a 'moral sense' that tells us what is right and wrong? What difficulties are there in thinking this?

8. 'Rule-utilitarianism is no more than a disguised form of act-utilitarianism, with all the same old problems.' Discuss.

9. Is it wrong to deceive a man engaged in criminal activity?

10. Read the following extract. What are the problems involved? How would Kant, Ross, and the rule-utilitarians deal with them?

> When I was a fourth-year student, William Sidney Thayer – the great professor at Hopkins, that wonderful understanding warm human being – came to Harvard and gave a Care of the Patient lecture. He described malignant disease and told how you handled it and how you always had to tell the patient the truth. This was a vivid experience for me. He described a patient who had come to him in Baltimore because he had been put off by physicians elsewhere. He knew he wasn't getting the answer, and so it was easy, I suppose, for Dr Thayer to know that the thing to do was to tell him. The patient wanted it; that was why he came to Baltimore. So he told him. The fellow, of course, was upset; and his wife was angry with Dr Thayer. He said she berated him; 'What right did you have to tell him?' Then, two hours later, he got a telephone call. They had gone back to their hotel, and called Dr Thayer to thank him for having told, because for the first time in several months, the two of them could sit down and talk.
>
> That was a vivid model, and now I think of my mistakes. A woman had obvious cancer of the thyroid, and knew it. She knew it because of the way her physician dodged telling her; everybody was alarmed. Any fool could see that her doctors were alarmed; so she made me promise the night before the operation, religiously promise, that I would tell her the truth. She suspected the truth; she outlined to me the number of reasons she needed to know. She was a widow; her children were not quite launched and so on; and I had to tell her for very practical reasons. So it was. It was a rapidly growing, undifferentiated carcinoma, the type with a wretched prognosis, perhaps nine months or a year, and it would have to be treated by radiation.
>
> So I waited until she was over the anaesthetic, and the next morning I came in, pulled up a chair next to her, sat down by her bedside, and said: 'I will now do what you asked me to do. You have a serious condition: we are going to give you X-ray treatment. There is no doubt that these treatments will help you. It is possible we will manage to eliminate the trouble completely, but just the same you had better do what you said about rearranging your estate and taking care of your children and so on.' She thanked me very much, and I went out with great relief, thinking that I had carried it off. In the next two or three days, I was congratulating myself because she had taken it so well; I must have done a good job. On the

fourth postoperative day, the nurse stopped me before I entered the room. 'You know, Mrs B is waiting. She wants to know when you are going to fulfil your promise and tell her what you found.' I was younger then than I am now; I failed to take advantage of the broad hint offered me by the patient, namely, that she had shut out the bad news. So I went in and I said, 'I hear from your nurse that I haven't told you. Don't you recall that the very day after the operation I told you?' 'Told me what?' So I went over it again. She, of course, went into a serious depression; and it was terrible. It ruined her life and, what is more, mistakes seem to be contagious. To make a long story short, the pathologist and I thought this was an undifferentiated carcinoma. It wasn't; it was one of those very peculiar tumors. The same type of tumor was found in the wall of her stomach four years later. She lived for 12 years after that to die of a coronary.[15]

Bibliography

1) The Ethical Theory of Immanuel Kant

* denotes text extracted in main text

Acton, H B *Kant's Moral Philosophy*, London, Macmillan, 1970.

Aune, Bruce *Kant's Theory of Morals*, Princeton, NJ: Princeton University Press, 1979

Cope, Oliver M *Man, Mind, and Machine*,* Philadelphia: J B Lippincott, 1968.

Glickman, Jack (ed.) *Moral Philosophy: An Introduction*, New York, St Martin's Press, 1976. An anthology of articles on Kantian ethics.

Gregor, Mary J *Laws of Freedom: A Study of Kant's Method of Applying the Categorical Imperative in the Metaphysik der Sitten*, Oxford, Basil Blackwell, 1963.

Hill, Thomas 'Humanity as an End in Itself,' *Ethics*, 91, 1980-81, pp.84-99

Kant, I *Groundword of the Metaphysic of Morals*,* translated, with analysis and notes, by J J Paton in *The Moral Law*, London, Hutchinson & Co., 1972.

– *Kant on the Foundation of Morality*, Bloomington & London, Indiana University Press, 1970. A modern version of the *Groundwork*, translated with a commentary by B E A Liddell.

– *Lectures on Ethics*, trans Louis Infield, New York, Harper & Row, 1963.

Kemp, John *The Philosophy of Kant*, Oxford, Oxford University Press, 1979. Ch 3.

Korner, S *Kant*, Harmondsworth, Penguin Books, 1955.

Paton, H J *The Categorical Imperative*, London, Hutchinson's University Library, 1946. A detailed account of Kant's moral philosophy.

Ross, W D *Kant's Ethical Theory*, Oxford, Oxford University Press, 1954.

Seneca, Lucius Annaeus *Epistulae Morales*, Vol 2, trans. Richard M Gummere, London, William Heinemann, 1970. pp 57-59.

Tomlin, E W F *The Western Philosophers*, London, Hutchinson & Co, 1968. pp 197-214.

Walker, Ralph C S *Kant*, London, Routledge & Kegal Paul, 1978. Ch 11.

15. Oliver M. Cope, *Man, Mind, and Machine*, Philadelphia, J.B. Lippincott, 1968, pp.28-29.

Ward, Keith *The Development of Kant's View of Ethics*, Oxford, Basil Blackwell, 1972) Ch 7 contains a clear exposition of the Groundwork.

Williams, Bernard *Ethics and the Limits of Philosophy*, London, Collins, 1985. Especially Ch 4.

Williams, T C *The Concept of the Categorical Imperative*, Oxford, Clarendon Press, 1968. An account of various interpretations of Kant's moral theory.

2) Some Criticisms and Amendments of Kant

Ewing, A C *Ethics*, London, The English Universities Press, 1969. Excellent chapters on Kant and Ross (and Moore).

Lyons, David *Forms and Limits of Utilitarianism*, Oxford, Clarendon Press, 1964. A difficult book, questioning the validity of the distinction between act- and rule-utilitarianism.

Narveson, J *Morality and Utility*, Baltimore, Maryland, The Johns Hopkins Press, 1967. Ch 4 on rule-utilitarianism.

Nowell-Smith, Patrick *Ethics*, Baltimore, Pelican Books, 1954. Especially Ch 16.

Ross, W D *The Right and the Good*, * Oxford, Oxford University Press, 1930.

Singer, Marcus *Generalization in Ethics*, New York, Random House, 1961. An influential book, arguing that universalization (or generalization) is the fundamental, but not the only, principle required by morality.

'The Golden Rule,' *The Encyclopedia of Philosophy*, ed. Paul Edwards, New York, Macmillan, 1967, III, pp.365-367.

Smart, J J C *Outlines of a Utilitarian System of Ethics*, London, Cambridge University Press, 1961. A powerful defence of rule-utilitarianism.

Chapter Seven
Discussion: Kant and the
Ethics of Truth-telling

THE DUTY OF TRUTH

As we saw in the last question of the previous chapter, one of the most persistent moral dilemmas faced by health professionals is: Should I tell my patients the truth? The usual presumption is, of course, that truth-telling is a moral good and that lying is a moral evil; but it is not difficult to imagine situations in which this distinction does not deal with the actual situations in which doctors and nurses sometimes find themselves. Should this patient be told that his drugs have unpleasant side-effects? Should the wife be told of her husband's HIV infection? Should a nine-year-old boy be told that he has inoperable cancer? Are there, in other words, circumstances in which a patient's right to know the truth about himself may not be in his best interests, and in which the doctor may best serve his patient by lying to him? Are there, then, occasions when telling the truth may do more harm than good, when a deliberate falsehood discharges another duty of care: 'First, do no harm' (the Hippocratic principle: *primum non nocere*)?

As a strict deontologist Kant's position is quite clear. Telling the truth, no matter what the consequences may be for oneself or for others, is an absolute duty of the will. Kant, therefore, can envisage no circumstances in which this duty can be abrogated. As he says, 'Truthfulness in statements which cannot be avoided is the formal duty of an individual to everyone, however great may be the disadvantage accruing to himself or to another.'[1] This follows, we remember, from the demands of the categorical imperative and the principle of universalizability which require us to act in such a way that 'my maxim should become a universal law.' Lying, indeed, is one of the examples Kant gives of the irrationality of what he calls a *contradiction in the law of nature.* Lying cannot be consistently universalised because to do so would undermine the practice of truth-telling upon which lying depends.[2]

It is no use, then, claiming that some lies are benevolent, that there may be, after all, certain lies that are excusable because they prevent harm and do good. For Kant all lying is wrong. He gives an example. How am I to answer the murderer's question about the whereabouts of his intended victim? Kant's reply is that, even here, one must tell the truth. The murder is someone else's crime, not yours; and if the crime follows from your telling the truth, one cannot be held responsible for the consequences. If, on the other hand, one lies, then one does become responsible for what subsequently happens. I might say, for instance, that the person sought was somewhere else, only to find to my horror that I had inadvertently given away his hiding-place. Then indeed I

---

1. Quoted by Sissela Bok, *Lying: Moral Choice in Public and Private Life*, Hassocks, Sussex, The Harvester Press, 1978, p. 38.
2. See above, p. 106

have become implicated in the crime. But no blame can attach to me for speaking the truth. For truth-telling, Kant tells us, is not a matter of expediency but an absolute imperative of morality, a categoric obligation imposed on me, irrespective of the particular situation in which I might find myself.

I think it is fair to say that most people find this inflexible position very hard to sustain and agree that there are occasions when telling a lie is morally justifiable. For W D Ross, we remember, the duty to tell the truth should be considered a *prima facie* duty, as an obligation which can be overridden by another and more compelling prima facie duty.[3] In the case just cited, for example, I may believe that lying to the murderer is justified by my earlier promise to the victim (the duty of fidelity) or by what I already owe him (the duty of gratitude). I may also believe that my priority in this instance lies in seeing that no harm comes to him (the duty of nonmalificence) or that virtue is best served by refusing the criminal's demands (the duty of beneficence). Either way, these possibilities reveal that the duty to speak the truth cannot be so rigorously and unimaginatively applied and that all our duties, although we may consider them laudable in themselves, will admit of exceptions.

Rule-utilitarians adopt a very similar position, albeit for rather different reasons. Lacking a concept of prima facie duty, the resolution of a conflict of interest lies not so much in juxtaposing one duty with another but in trying to estimate the particular consequences if everyone obeyed the same rule in a similar situation. Rule-utilitarians, in other terms, retain Kant's notion of universalizability but subject it to the utilitarian principle of utility. A rule is thus assessed in terms of whether its universal adoption would or would not maximise happiness. The fact, therefore, that 'telling the truth' is, in Kantian terms, a categorical imperative does not of itself require that it should always be obeyed. A doctor, for example, may lie to a badly-injured mother about the survival of her young son in the car crash, and justify his deception on the grounds that it increases her own immediate chances of survival. This, then, is an instance in which the obligation to tell the truth cannot be regarded as an absolute duty because here its observance produces adverse rather than beneficial effects.

AUTONOMY AND PATERNALISM

There is, however, another aspect of Kant's argument that should not be overlooked. We recall that one version of the categorical imperative insists that individuals should be treated 'never simply as a means, but always at the same time as an end.'[4] This requirement follows from Kant's view that human beings are creatures capable of rational thought, capable of understanding, for example, the universality of the moral law and of thereafter freely submitting themselves to its demands. Men and women are, to use Kant's important term, **autonomous** beings: they are motivated to act morally not through inclination, still less through coercion, but through their own perception of their duty in accordance with universal law. For one human being not to respect another's

3. See above, p. 112
4. See above, p. 107

autonomy – to treat him merely 'as a means' – is therefore to deny to another the respect that should be his as a self-ruling, independent and rational agent. That such a denial is immoral is clearly evidenced by the fact that it produces a *contradiction in the will*. The assertion of my autonomy to the exclusion of others would result, if universalised, in the denial of my own autonomy by others, and this no rational human being could desire.

Recognition of the principle that man is an end in himself provides us with a further argument against ever telling lies. Lying is a denial of autonomy and thus is a form of exploitation of man by man. With the lie, in other words, one individual, however well-intentioned, deprives another of the right to exercise a free choice in his own affairs. In deliberately withholding information from this patient, the doctor is therefore interfering with the autonomous process of decision-making, and thus debasing his patient to the level of a mere 'means'. But it is not for the doctor to adjudicate on whether the truth is better left unsaid, since truth-telling is a duty owed by doctor to his patient as one autonomous individual to another. Truth-telling, as Kant would have it, is an instance of the good will at work: it is an imperative of morality and as such can incur no blame, not even if it brings suffering and grief in its wake.

Even in this new version, the rigidity of Kant's position is quite apparent and gives little assistance in those situations where the patient may lack the capacity to be autonomous. One thinks, for instance, of those who are unconscious, infirm, mentally disabled or too frightened or too young to understand their situation. In these cases, many would argue, it is morally right for the physician to take on the responsibility of decision-making, and to allow his own technical expertise to take precedence over those with impaired autonomy. The doctor does not, then, deceive his patient out of a lack regard for him as an autonomous being but because he believes the patient will be best served if he is treated as a 'means to an end' – the end being here the patient's own recovery. In these circumstances lying may be deemed an *instrumental good*: not a good in itself but the means of achieving a beneficent result. The model relationship usually cited here is that between a father and a son. The father, we agree, has the right to restrict his child's freedom in various ways – and, if need be, to be evasive and deceitful in the process – if this results in the removal of the child from situations of danger. This is the model known as benevolent **paternalism** (or 'parentalism'). By the same token, and as an instance of medical paternalism, the doctor has the right to remove his patient from danger, and if necessary to employ similar forms of evasion and deception to achieve this, regardless of whether the patient recognises that he is at risk, regardless of whether he has consented to the proposed form of treatment, and regardless of whether the patient knows of the likely consequences and of the availability of alternative treatments.

Paternalism has been defined by Gerald Dworkin as the 'interference with a person's liberty of action justified by reasons referring exclusively to the welfare, good, happiness, needs, interests or values of the person coerced.'[5] This well-known definition, however, needs further explanation. According to Joel Feinberg, we should make two additional distinctions.[6] We should first distinguish between paternalism that seeks a) to protect the individual from harm, and b) to bring about the individual's own good. Each of these forms can then be further divided into two types, the 'weak' and the 'strong'.

In **weak paternalism** a person is, by and large, committed to the prevention of harm (and the promotion of good) when he believes that the harm arises from conduct that is either substantially nonvoluntary (e.g. preventing an hallucinating drug addict from throwing himself out of a window), or ignorant or uninformed of its own consequences (e.g. preventing someone from ingesting a poisonous substance), or when that person feels it is necessary to act, if only temporarily, to establish whether the conduct is voluntary or not (e.g. snatching the woman away from the path of the oncoming bus). In essence, then, weak paternalism approves of interfering when the harm results from a lack of choice or lack of knowledge. In **strong paternalism** intervention to prevent harm (and to promote the good) is permitted when the harm results from an action that is both voluntary and informed. Governments, it may be argued, frequently act in this fashion. Laws and regulations concerning the wearing of seat-belts, smoking in public places, drinking and driving, carrying weapons and so on, may all be construed as preventative measures introduced precisely in order to protect the individual from the injuries accruing from his own voluntary choices. When we turn to more technical areas, like medicine, the paternalistic argument is still more persuasive. A well-known example here would be the case of a doctor overruling the religious convictions of a Jehovah's Witness and forcing him to have a blood transfusion. In this case the doctor's utilitarian concern to produce the greatest happiness overrides any respect he may otherwise have had for the patient's autonomy. If he further believes that suffering can be reduced by discarding the normal moral constraints of promise-keeping and truth-telling, then so be it.

In the following extracts, the tension between a patient's autonomous right to know the truth and the doctor's paternalistic right to withhold information is graphically demonstrated. In her well-known book on *Lying*, Sissela Bok attacks the idea that deceiving patients is justified on the teleological grounds of beneficial results. Not only is it by no means certain that patients do not want bad news but there is also little evidence to suggest that the truth will harm them. Rather the reverse in fact, if the deception, although perhaps laudable in intention, only serves to damage the trust upon which a good doctor-patient relationship in based. As a case in point, Bok examines the frequent and costly use of placebos in medicine, a practice which, she believes, only serves to undermine effective treatment and to perpetuate drug dependency.

Bok's position is challenged by Mack Lipkin. Lipkin's argument is based on his own practical experience as a physician. He claims that doctors are justified in deceiving their patients, or at least in withholding the truth from them, because telling them the whole truth is a 'practical impossibility.' He gives two reasons why this is the case: first, patients do not have sufficient

---

5. Gerald Dworkin, 'Paternalism', *Monist*, LV1, No.1, June 1972, p.65.
6. 'Legal Paternalism,' *Canadian Journal of Philosophy*, I, No.1, 1971, pp. 105-124. Reprinted in Feinberg, *Rights, Justice, and the Bounds of Liberty*, Princeton University Press, 1980, pp. 110-129.

medical knowledge to interpret the information accurately; and second, they frequently do not want to know the truth about their condition. For Lipkin, the only guiding principle to be employed here is whether the deception – such as a placebo – is intended to benefit the patient or the doctor.

In the third extract Grant Gillett tackles the question of truth-telling from a different perspective, and considers the problem of medical confidentiality. What should a doctor do if his patient refuses to tell his wife that he has AIDS? Should the doctor take it upon himself to disclose the truth or should he respect his patient's wishes and keep silent? Gillett considers the options from deontological and utilitarian points of view, and concludes that, in this instance, confidentiality can be suspended on the grounds that it is a *prima facie* duty, and so one that can be outweighed by other duties – in this case, the duty to see that no harm comes to any other person. The patient, indeed, by demanding silence, has shown a manifest disregard for the suffering of others and has thus placed himself outside the 'moral community' in which rules of confidentiality apply.

Extract 1: Sissela Bok: Placebos[7]

The common practice of prescribing placebos to unwitting patients illustrates the two miscalculations so common to minor forms of deceit: ignoring possible harm and failing to see how gestures assumed to be trivial build up into collectively undesirable practices.[8] Placebos have been used since the beginning of medicine. They can be sugar pills, salt-water injections – in fact, any medical procedure which has no specific effect on a patient's condition, but which can have powerful psychological effects leading to relief from symptoms such as pain or depression.

Placebos are prescribed with great frequency. Exactly how often cannot be known, the less so as physicians do not ordinarily talk publicly about using them. At times, self-deception enters in on the part of physicians, so that they have unwarranted faith in the powers of what can work only as a placebo. As with salesmanship, medication often involves unjustified belief in the excellence of what is suggested to others. In the past, most remedies were of a kind that, unknown to the medical profession and their patients, could have only placebic benefits, if any.

The derivation of 'placebo,' from the Latin for 'I shall please,' gives the word a benevolent ring, somehow placing placebos beyond moral criticism and conjuring up images of hypochondriacs whose vague ailments are dispelled through adroit prescriptions of beneficent sugar pills. Physicians often give a humorous tinge to instructions for prescribing these substances, which helps to remove them from serious ethical concern. . . . After all, health professionals argue, are not placebos far less dangerous than some genuine drugs? And more likely to produce a cure than if nothing at all is prescribed? . . .

Such a simplistic view conceals the real costs of placebos, both to individuals and to the practice of medicine. First, the resort to placebos may actually prevent the treatment of an underlying, undiagnosed problem. And even if the placebo 'works,' the effect is often shortlived; the symptoms may recur, or crop up in other

7. *Lying: Moral Choice in Public and Private Life*, Hassocks, Sussex, The Harvester Press, 1978, pp.61-68.
8. This discussion draws on my two articles, 'Paternalistic Deception in Medicine, and Rational Choice: The Use of Placebos,' in Max Black, ed., *Problems of Choice and Decision*, Ithaca. N.Y., Cornell University Program on Science, Technology and Society, 19 75, pp.73-107; and 'The Ethics of Giving Placebos,' *Scientific American*, 231, 1974, pp.17-23.

forms. Very often, the symptoms of which the patient complains are bound to go away by themselves, sometimes even from the mere contact with a health professional. In those cases, the placebo itself is unnecessary; having recourse to it merely reinforces a tendency to depend upon pills or treatments where none is needed.

In the aggregate, the costs of placebos are immense. Many millions of dollars are expended on drugs, diagnostic tests, and psychotherapies of a placebic nature. Even operations can be of this nature – a hysterectomy may thus be performed, not because the condition of the patient requires such surgery, but because she goes from one doctor to another seeking to have the surgery performed, or because she is judged to have a great fear of cancer which might be alleviated by the very fact of the operation.

Even apart from financial and emotional costs and the squandering of resources, the practice of giving placebos is wasteful of a very precious good: the trust on which so much in the medical relationship depends. The trust of those patients who find out they have been duped is lost, sometimes irretrievably. They may then lose confidence in physicians and even in bona fide medication which they may need in the future. They may obtain for themselves more harmful drugs or attach their hopes to debilitating fad cures. . . .

The patients who do *not* discover the deception and are left believing that a placebic remedy has worked may continue to rely on it under the wrong circumstances. This is especially true with drugs such as antibiotics, which are sometimes used as placebos and sometimes for their specific action. Many parents, for example, come to believe that they must ask for the prescription of antibiotics every time their child has a fever or a cold. The fact that so many doctors accede to such requests perpetuates the dependence of these families on medical care they do not need and weakens their ability to cope with health problems. Worst of all, those children who cannot tolerate antibiotics may have severe reactions, sometimes fatal, to such unnecessary medication.[9]

Such deceptive practices, by their very nature, tend to escape the normal restraints of accountability and can therefore spread more easily than others. There are many instances in which an innocuous-seeming practice has grown to become a large-scale and more dangerous one. Although warnings against the 'entering wedge' are often rhetorical devices, they can at times express justifiable caution; especially when there are great pressures to move along the undesirable path and when the safeguards are insufficient.

In this perspective, there is much reason for concern about placebos. The safeguards against this practice are few or nonexistent – both because it is secretive in nature and because it is condoned but rarely carefully discussed in the medical literature.[10] And the pressures are very great, and growing stronger, from drug companies, patients eager for cures, and busy physicians, for more medication, whether it is needed or not. Given this lack of safeguards and these strong pressures, the use of placebos can spread in a number of ways.

The clearest danger lies in the gradual shift from pharmacologically inert placebos to more active ones. It is not always easy to distinguish completely inert substances from somewhat active ones and these in turn from more active ones. It may be hard to distinguish between a quantity of an active substance so low that it has little or no effect and quantities that have some effect. It is not always clear to doctors whether patients require an inert placebo or possibly a more active

9. C M Kunin, T Tupasi, & W Craig, 'Use of Antibiotics,' *Annals of Internal Medicine*, 79, Oct. 1973, pp.555-60.
10. In a sample of nineteen recent, often used textbooks, in medicine, paediatrics, surgery, anaesthesia, obstetrics, and gynaecology, only three even mention placebos, none detail either medical or ethical dilemmas they pose. Four out of six textbooks on pharmacology mention them; only one mentions such problems. Only four out of eight textbooks on psychiatry mention placebos; none takes up ethical problems. For references, see Bok, 'Paternalistic Deception in Medicine and Rational Choice.'

one, and there can be the temptation to resort to an active one just in case it might also have a specific effect. It is also much easier to deceive a patient with a medication that is known to be 'real' and to have power. One recent textbook in medicine goes so far as to advocate the use of small doses of effective compounds as placebos rather than inert substances – because it is important for both the doctor and the patient to believe in the treatment! This shift is made easier because the dangers and side effects of active agents are not always known or considered important by the physician.

Meanwhile, the number of patients receiving placebos increases as more and more people seek and receive medical care and as their desire for instant, push-button alleviation of symptoms is stimulated by drug advertising and by rising expectations of what science can do. The use of placebos for children grows as well, and the temptations to manipulate the truth are less easily resisted once such great inroads have already been made.

Deception by placebo can be spread from therapy and diagnosis to experimentation. Much experimentation with placebos is honest and consented to by the experimental subjects, especially since the advent of strict rules governing such experimentation. But grievous abuses have taken place where placebos were given to unsuspecting subjects who believed they had received another substance. In 1971, for example, a number of Mexican-American women applied to a family-planning clinic for contraceptives. Some of them were given oral contraceptives and others were given placebos, or dummy pills that looked like the real thing. Without fully informed consent, the women were being used in an experiment to explore the side effects of various contraceptive pills. Some of those who were given placebos experienced a predictable side effect – they became pregnant. The investigators neither assumed financial responsibility for the babies nor indicated any concern about having bypassed the 'informed consent' that is required in ethical experiments with human beings. One contented himself with the observation that if only the law had permitted it, he could have aborted the pregnant women!

The failure to think about the ethical problems in such a case stems at least in part from the innocent-seeming white lies so often told in giving placebos. The spread from therapy to experimentation and from harmlessness to its opposite often goes unnoticed in part *because* of the triviality believed to be connected with placebos as white lies. This lack of foresight and concern is most frequent when the subjects in the experiment are least likely to object or defend themselves; as with the poor, the institutionalised, and the very young.

In view of all these ways in which placebo usage can spread, it is not enough to look at each incident of manipulation in isolation, no matter how benevolent it may be. When the costs and benefits are weighed, not only the individual conse-quences must be considered, but also the cumulative ones. Reports of deceptive practices inevitably leak out, and the resulting suspicion is heightened by the anxiety which threats to health always create. And so even the health profession-als who do not mislead their patients are injured by those who do; the entire institution of medicine is threatened by practices lacking in candor, however harm-less the results may appear in some individual cases.

This is not to say that all placebos must be ruled out; merely that they cannot be excused as innocuous. They should be prescribed but rarely, and only after a careful diagnosis and consideration of non-deceptive alternatives; they should be used in experimentation only after subjects have consented to their use.

Extract 2: Mack Lipkin: On Lying to Patients[11]

Should a doctor always tell his patients the truth? In recent years there has been an extraordinary increase in public discussion of the ethical problems involved in this question. But little has been heard from physicians themselves. I believe that gaps in understanding the complex interactions between doctors and patients have led many laymen astray in this debate.

It is easy to make an attractive case for always telling patients the truth. But as L. J. Henderson, the great Harvard physiologist-philosopher of decades ago, commented:

> To speak of telling the truth, the whole truth and nothing but the truth to a patient is absurd. Like absurdity in mathematics, it is absurd simply because it is impossible. . . . The notion that the truth, the whole truth, and nothing but the truth can be conveyed to the patient is a good specimen of that class of fallacies called by Whitehead 'the fallacy of misplaced concreteness.' It results from neglecting factors that cannot be excluded from the concrete situation and that are of an order of magnitude and relevancy that make it imperative to consider them. Of course, another fallacy is also often involved, the belief that diagnosis and prognosis are more certain than they are. But that is another question.

Words, especially medical terms, inevitably carry different implications for different people. When these words are said in the presence of anxiety-laden illness, there is a strong tendency to hear selectively and with emphases not intended by the doctor. Thus, what the doctor means to convey is obscured.

Indeed, thoughtful physicians know that transmittal of accurate information to patients is often impossible. Patients rarely know how the body functions in health and disease, but instead have inaccurate ideas of what is going on; this hampers the attempts to 'tell the truth.'

Take cancer, for example. Patients seldom know that while some cancers are rapidly fatal, others never amount to much; some have a cure rate of 99 percent, others less than 1 percent; a cancer may grow rapidly for months and then stop growing for years; may remain localised for years or spread all over the body almost from the beginning; some can be arrested for long periods of time, others not. Thus, one patient thinks of cancer as curable, the next thinks it means certain death.

How many patients understand that 'heart trouble' may refer to literally hundreds of different abnormalities ranging in severity from the trivial to the instantly fatal? How many know that the term 'arthritis' may refer to dozens of different types of joint involvement? 'Arthritis' may raise a vision of the appalling disease that made Aunt Eulalee a helpless invalid until her death years later; the next patient remembers Grandpa grumbling about the damned arthritis as he got up from his chair. Unfortunately but understandably, most people's ideas about the implications of medical terms are based on what they have heard about a few cases.

The news of serious illness drives some patients to irrational and destructive behavior; others handle it sensibly. A distinguished philosopher forestalled my telling him about his cancer by saying, 'I want to know the truth. The only thing I couldn't take and wouldn't want to know about is cancer.' For two years he had watched his mother die slowly of a painful form of cancer. Several of my physician patients have indicated they would not want to know if they had a fatal illness.

Most patients should be told 'the truth' to the extent that they can comprehend it. Indeed, most doctors, like most other people, are uncomfortable with lies. Good physicians, aware that some may be badly damaged by being told more than they

11. *Newsweek*, 4 June 1979, p.13.

want or need to know, can usually ascertain the patient's preferences and needs.

Discussions about lying often center about the use of placebos. In medical usage, a 'placebo' is a treatment that has no specific physical or chemical action on the condition being treated, but is given to affect symptoms by a psychologic mechanism, rather than a purely physical one. Ethicists believe that placebos necessarily involve a partial or complete deception by the doctor, since the patient is allowed to believe that the treatment has a specific effect. They seem unaware that placebos, far from being inert (except in the rigid pharmacological sense), are among the most powerful agents known to medicine.

Placebos are a form of suggestion, which is a direct or indirect presentation of an idea, followed by an uncritical, i.e. not thought-out, acceptance. Those who have studied suggestion or looked at medical history know its almost unbelievable potency; it is involved to a greater or lesser extent in the treatment of every conscious patient. It can induce or remove almost any kind of feeling or thought. It can strengthen the weak or paralyze the strong; transform sleeping, feeding, or sexual patterns; remove or induce a vast array of symptoms; mimic or abolish the effect of very powerful drugs. It can alter the function of most organs. It can cause illness or a great sense of well-being. It can kill. In fact, doctors often add a measure of suggestion when they prescribe even potent medications for those who also need psychologic support. Like all potent agents, its proper use requires judgment based on experience and skill.

Communication between physician and the apprehensive and often confused patient is delicate and uncertain. Honesty should be evaluated not only in terms of a slavish devotion to language often misinterpreted by the patient, but also in terms of intent. *The crucial question is whether the deception was intended to benefit the patient or the doctor.*

Physicians, like most people, hope to see good results and are disappointed when patients do poorly. Their reputations and their livelihood depend on doing effective work; purely selfish reasons would dictate they do their best for their patients. Most important, all good physicians have a deep sense of responsibility toward those who have entrusted their welfare to them.

As I have explained, it is usually a practical impossibility to tell patients 'the whole truth.' Moreover, often enough, the ethics of the situation, the true moral responsibility, may demand that the naked facts not be revealed. The now popular complaint that doctors are too authoritarian is misguided more often than not. Some patients who insist on exercising their right to know may be doing themselves a disservice.

Judgment is often difficult and uncertain. Simplistic assertions about telling the truth may not be helpful to parents or physicians in times of trouble.

Extract 3: Grant Gillett: AIDS and Confidentiality[12]

Does a doctor confronted by a patient with AIDS have a duty to maintain absolute confidentiality or could that doctor be considered to have some overriding duty to the sexual contacts of the AIDS sufferer? AIDS or Acquired Immune Deficiency is a viral disease transmitted for the most part by sexual contact. It is fatal in the short or long term (i.e. nine months to six years) in those infected people who go on to develop the full-blown form of the disease.

Let us say that a 39 year old man goes to his family doctor with a dry persistent cough which has lasted three or four weeks and a 10 day history of night sweats. He admits that he is bisexually active. He is tested and found to have antibodies

12. *Journal of Applied Philosophy*, IV, No.1 (1987) pp.15-20.

to HIV virus (indicating that he is infected with the virus that causes AIDS). In the setting of this clinical picture he must be considered to have the disease. He is told of his condition and also, in the course of a prolonged interview, of the risk to his wife and of the distinct possibility of his children aged one and three years old being left without parents should she contract the disease. He refuses to allow her to be told of his condition. The doctor finally accedes to his demand for absolute confidentiality. After one or two initial illnesses which are successfully combatted he dies some 18 months later. Over the last few weeks of his life he relents on his former demands and allows his wife to be informed of his problem. She is tested and, though asymptomatic, is found to be antibody positive. A year later she goes to the doctor with fever, dry cough and loss of appetite. Distraught on behalf of her children, she bitterly accuses the doctor of having failed her and them by allowing her husband to infect her when steps could have been taken to diminish the risk had she only known the truth.

In this case there is a powerful inclination to say that the wife is justified in her grievance. It seems just plain wrong for her doctor to sit back and allow her to fall victim to a fatal disease because of the wish of her husband. Against this intuition we can mobilise two powerful arguments – one deontological and the other utilitarian (of a rule or restricted utilitarian type).

(i) On a deontological view the practice of medicine will be guided by certain inviolate or absolute rules (not to harm, not to neglect the welfare of one's patients, etc.). Among these will be respect for confidentiality. Faced with this inviolable principle the deontologically inclined physician will not disclose what he has been told in confidence – he will regard the tacit agreement not to disclose his patient's affairs to others as tantamount to a substantive promise which he cannot break. Against this, in the present case, we might urge his *prima facie* duty not to neglect the welfare of his other patient, the young man's wife. His inaction has contributed to her death. In response to this he could both defend the absolute duty to respect confidentiality in general and urge some version of the doctrine of double effect, claiming that his clear duty was to honour his implicit vow of confidentiality but it had the unfortunate effect, which he had foreseen as possible but not intended, that it caused the death of his other patient. One is inclined to offer an intuitive response such as 'No moral duty is so binding that you can hazard another person's life in this manner.' It is a notorious feature of deontological systems that they involve conflicts of duties for which there exists no principled method of resolution.

(ii) A rule-utilitarian doctor can mount a more convincing case. He can observe that confidentiality is a cornerstone of a successful AIDS practice. Lack of confidentiality can cause the irrational victimisation of sufferers by a poorly educated public who are prone to witch-hunts of all kinds. The detection and treatment of AIDS, and the consequent protection of that large group of people who have contacts with the patients being treated depends on the patients who seek medical advice believing that medical confidentiality is inviolate. If confidentiality were seen as a relative duty only, suspended or breached at the discretion of the doctor, then far fewer cases would present for detection and crucial guidance about diminishing risks of spread would not be obtained. This would lead to more people suffering and dying. It may be hard on a few, unfortunate enough to be involved with people like the recalcitrant young husband, but the general welfare can only be served by a compassionate but resolute refusal to abandon sound principles in the face of such cases. Many find this a convincing argument but I will argue that it is superficial in the understanding of moral issues that it espouses. . . .

Imagine, in order to soften the way for a rather less neatly argued position, a doctor confronted by a young man who has a scratched face and blood on his shirt and who wants to be checked for VD. In the course of the doctor's taking his history it emerges that he has forcibly raped two women and is worried that the second was a prostitute. He says to the doctor 'Of course, I am telling you this in confidence, doc, because I know that you won't rat on me.' Producing a knife, he then says, 'See, this is the blade that I get them going with.' Rather troubled, the doctor takes samples and tells the young man that there is no evidence of VD. He tries to talk his patient into giving himself up for some kind of psychiatric treatment but the young man is adamant. It becomes clear that he has certain delusional and persecutional ideas. Two days later the doctor reads that his patient has been arrested because after leaving the surgery he raped and savagely mutilated a young woman who, as a result, required emergency surgery for multiple wounds and remains in a critical condition.

Here we might well feel that any principle which dictates that it is the moral duty of the doctor to keep silent is wrong – but as yet no principles conflicting with or supplementing those above have been introduced. A possible loophole is introduced by the rapist's sadomasochism and probable psychosis but we need to spell out why this is relevant. In such a case we suspend our normal moral obligations to respect the avowed interests of the patient and claim that he is incompetent to make a responsible and informed assessment of his own interests and so we assume the right to make certain decisions on his behalf. . . . He is insane because a normal person would never begin from the moral position he occupies and so his rights, including that to medical confidentiality, are suspended. He has moved outside the community of trust, mutual concern and non-malificence in which moral considerations for the preferences of others have their proper place. . . . We are, of course, not released from a *prima facie* duty to try and help him in his odious predicament but we cannot be expected to accord him the full privileges of a member of the moral community as he persists, for whatever reason, in callously turning his back on the constraints normally operative there (albeit, perhaps, without reflective malevolence in its more usual forms). So, in this case, confidentiality can be suspended for legitimate moral reasons. . . .

We can now move from a case where insanity weights the decision in a certain direction to a case where the issues are more purely moral. Imagine that a 45-year-old man goes to see his family doctor and is also worried about a sexually transmitted disease. On being questioned he admits, in confidence, not only to intercourse with a series of prostitutes but also to forced sexual intercourse with his daughter. He is confident that she will not tell anyone what is happening because she is too ashamed and scared. After counselling he gives no sign of a wish to change his ways but rather continues to justify himself because of his wife's behaviour. The doctor later hears from the school psychological service that the daughter is showing some potentially serious emotional problems.

Here, it seems to me, we have few compunctions about setting in motion that machinery to deal with child abuse, even though the sole source of our information is what was said, in medical confidence, by the father. The justification we might give for the doctor's actions is illuminating. We are concerned for the actual harm being done to the child, both physical and psychological, and we overturn the father's injunction to confidence in order to prevent further harm being done. In so doing we class the situation as one in which a *prima facie* moral claim can be suspended because of the actions and attitudes involved. I believe that we do so because we implicitly realise that here also the agent has acted in such a way as to put himself beyond the full play of moral consideration and to justify our witholding certain of his moral 'dues'. Confidentiality functions to allow the patient to be honest with the doctor and to put trust in him. The legitimate expectation that a doctor be trustworthy and faithful to his patient's wishes regardless of the behaviour of that patient is undermined when the patient abuses the relationship so formed in ways which show a lack of these basic human reactions because it is just these reactions which ground the importance of confidentiality in general. Therefore, if the father in this example refuses to accept the enormity of what he is doing to his daughter, he thereby casts doubt upon his standing as a moral agent. Stated baldly, that sounds like an open warrant for moralistic medical paternalism, but I do not think it need be. In asking that his affairs be concealed from others, a person is demanding *either* the right to preserve himself from the harms that might befall him if the facts about his life were generally known, *or* that his sensitivity as an individual be respected and protected. On either count it is inconsistent for him to claim some moral justification for that demand when it is made solely with the aim of allowing him to inflict comparable disregard or harm upon another. By his implicit intention to use a position, which only remains tenable with the collusion of the doctor, callously to harm another individual, the father undermines the moral force of his own appeal. His case is only worsened by the fact that from any moral perspective he would be considered to have a special and protective obligation toward his own offspring. . . .

Implicit within what I have said is a reappraisal of the nature of medical confidentiality. I have argued that it is not to be treated as an absolute duty but is rather to rank among other *prima facie* duties and responsibilities of the doctor-patient relationship. Just as the performance of a life-saving procedure can be vetoed by the patient's choice to forego treatment, even though it is a doctor's duty to strive for his patient's life, so each of these duties can be negated by certain considerations. One generally attempts to prevent a fatal illness overtaking a patient but in the case of a deformed neonate or an elderly and demented patient often the attempt is not made. In the case of confidentiality, I have claimed that we recognise the right of a patient to preserve his own personal life as inviolate. We accept that patients can and should share with a doctor details which it would not be right to disclose to other people. But we must also recognise that implicit within this recognition is the assumption that the patient is one of us, morally speaking. Our attitude to him and his rights assumes that he is one of or a participant in a community of beings who matter (or are morally interacting individuals like himself to whom the same considerations apply). We could offer a superficial and rather gross systematisation of this assumption in the universalizability test. The patient in the last two case applies a standard to his own human concerns which he is not prepared to extend to others involved with him in relevant situations. We must therefore regard his moral demands as spurious; we are not at liberty to harm him but we are bound to see that his cynical abuse of the moral code within which he lives does not harm others. . . .

Now we can return to the AIDS patient. From what I have said it becomes clear that it is only the moral intransigent who forces us to breach confidentiality. In most cases it will be possible to guide the patient into telling those who need to know or allowing them to be told (and where it is possible to so guide him it will be mandatory to involve him in an informed way). In the face of an expressed disregard for the harm being caused to those others concerned, we will be morally correct in abandoning what would otherwise be a binding obligation. We should and do feel the need to preserve and protect the already affected life of the potential victim of his deception and in this feeling we exhibit a sensitivity to moral rectitude. Of course, it is only the active sexual partners of the patient who are at risk and thus it is only to them that we and the patient have a moral duty (in this respect talk of 'society at large' is just rhetoric). . . .

The doctor's obligation to inform, in the face of an enjoinder to keep his confidence, can, even if I am right, be seen to be restricted to those in actual danger and would in no wise extend to employers, friends or non-sexually interacting relatives of the patient or any other person with an even more peripheral interest. His duty extends only so far as to avert the actual harm that he can reasonably expect to arise from his keeping confidence.

Given the intransigent case, one further desideratum presents itself. I believe that doctors should be open with their patients and that therefore the doctor is bound to share his moral dilemma with the patient and inform him of his intention to breach confidentiality. I think he can legitimately claim a pre-emptive duty to prevent harm befalling his patients and should do so in the case of the abuse of others which the patient intends. It may be the case, with the insane rapist for instance, that the doctor will need to deceive in order to carry out his prevailing duty but this will hardly ever be so, and should, I believe, be regarded as unacceptable in general.

One thorny problem remains – the possible deleterious effect on the detection and treatment of AIDS if confidentiality is seen as only a relative principle in medical practice. Clearly, if the attitude were ever to take root that the medical profession could not be trusted to 'keep their mouths shut' then the feared effect would occur. I believe that where agencies and informal groups were told of the *only* grounds on which confidentiality would be breached and the *only* people who would be informed then this effect would not occur. . . .

Questions

1. Is Kant right to argue that truthfulness can never do harm? Give examples from medical practice.

2. Is telling patients the truth an absolute duty or a *prima facie* duty? Consider this question when knowing the truth will decrease a patient's chances of recovery.

3. Is Lipkin right to claim that truth-telling is a 'practical impossibility'?

4. A patient asks, 'Doctor, will you tell me the truth?' In what circumstances would you deny him his request?

5. Does a doctor have a duty to obstruct a patient from pursuing a disastrous course of treatment? May the doctor resort to deception to achieve her ends?

6. Is the use of placebos ever justified?

7. In what circumstances is the health professional correct in treating his patient as a 'means to an end' ?

8. 'Neither one person, nor any number of persons, is warranted in saying to another human creature of ripe years, that he shall not do with his life for his own benefit what he chooses to do with it.' (Mill). Discuss.

9. Is the mutual trust between doctor and patient irreparably impaired if it begins with the doctor stating the conditions in which confidentiality may be broken? Give examples.

10. Consider the following case. Did the doctor act correctly or should he have respected his patient's confidentiality, come what may? Should the fact that the wife was not at risk have affected his decision?

> John was in his mid-thirties, married and with two young children, when his company sent him to set up a new branch in Central Africa. He was nine months on his own, and during that time he worked exceptionally hard and successfully, letting himself go only on one regretted occasion when, after a convivial evening with some clients, he visited a local brothel.
>
> By the time John returned home, Jane had found a cottage in her parents' village where their belongings could be stored when they returned to Africa together. To buy the cottage, John needed a small mortgage, and two questions on the form led him from Dr Browne, their family doctor, to a London consultant and back again. It was just good luck, Dr Browne told him, that Jane's gynaecological condition had temporarily prevented them from having intercourse since their return. But John now clearly had no alternative but to tell her that he was HIV-positive.
>
> John loved Jane, but knew her nature, part-Puritan, part-hypochondriac. When he came back to see Dr Browne after thinking things over, he tried to explain his misgivings about telling her. Dr Browne was unimpressed: John was like a man with a loaded revolver as far as his wife was concerned, he told him. He was also more explicit about his own potential role. His duty of confidentiality towards John was not absolute. Jane was also his patient; and both the General Medical Council and the British Medical Association made it clear that in these circumstances he could breach confidence.
>
> Reluctantly, John told Jane. As he feared, she took his confession extremely badly, becoming quite hysterical and refusing to listen further. She took the children home to her parents, saying that it was not safe for them to be in the same house as him, and shortly after she began divorce proceedings. Before he went back to Africa, John revisited the consultant in London, who discussed his options, gave him some good practical advice and told him how he might know when it was time to come back. When the time came however, unable to face his situation and the prospect of dying of AIDS, John killed himself.[13]

Bibliography

* denotes text extracted in main text

Ackerman, Terrence F 'Why Doctors Should Intervene,' *Hastings Center Report*, XII, August 1982, pp.14-17.

Beauchamp, Tom (with Laurence B McCullough) *Medical Ethics: The Moral Responsibilities of Physicians*, Englewood Cliffs, N.J., Prentice-Hall, 1984. A thorough analysis of the tension between seeking patient benefit and respecting his autonomy.

Bok, Sissela *Lying: Moral Choice in Public and Private Life,** Hassocks, Sussex, The Harvester Press, 1978

Childress, James F *Who Should Decide?: Paternalism in Health Care*, New York & Oxford, Oxford University Press, 1982

13. Kenneth M Boyd, 'HIV infection and AIDS: the ethics of medical confidentiality', *Journal of Medical Ethics*, XVIII (1992) p.174 (original pp. 173-179

– 'Paternalism and Health Care,' in *Medical Responsibility*, ed. Wade L Robison and Michael S Pritchard, New York, Humana Press, 1979, pp.15-27

Dworkin, Gerald 'Paternalism,' *Monist*, LVI, 1972, pp.64-84.

– *The Theory and Practice of Autonomy*, Cambridge, Cambridge University Press, 1988

Faden, Ruth R (with Tom L Beauchamp). *A History and Theory of Informed Consent*, New York, Oxford University Press, 1986). An exhaustive account of informed consent in various fields: medicine, philosophy and law.

Feinberg, Joel'Legal Paternalism,' *Canadian Journal of Philosophy*, 1, No.1, 1971, pp. 105-24. Reprinted in Feinberg, *Rights, Justice, and the Bounds of Liberty*, Princeton, Princeton University Press, 1980, pp.110-129.

Gillett, Grant 'Aids and Confidentiality,'* *Journal of Applied Philosophy*, IV, No.1, 1987, pp.15-20.

– *Reasonable Care*, Bristol, The Bristol Press, 1989.

Goldman, Alan H *The Moral Foundations of Professional Ethics*, Totowa, N.J., Littlefield, Adams & Co., 1980. Analyses when professional obligations should overrule the normal moral obligations.

Higgs, Roger 'On Telling Patients the Truth,' *Moral Dilemmas in Modern Medicine*, ed. Michael Lockwood, Oxford, Oxford University Press, pp.188-202.

– (ed.) 'A father says "Don't tell my son the truth,"' *Journal of Medical Ethics*, 11, 1985, pp.153-158. A case conference.

Kirk, Carol A van (with Edward D Schreck). 'Truth-telling and Placebos: A Conflict of Duties,' *Listening*, 22, 1987, pp.52-65. An interesting discussion, set in the context of Ross' ethical theory.

Kottow, Michael H 'Medical confidentiality: an intransigent and absolute obligation,' *Journal of Medical Ethics*, 12, pp.117-122.

Kübler-Ross, Elizabeth *On Death and Dying*, New York, Macmillan, 1969. A famous book, with an important section on the ethics of lying.

Lindley, Richard *Autonomy*, Atlantic Highlands, N. J., Humanities Press, 1986. Examines various concepts of autonomy and relates them to various social and medical problems.

Lipkin, Mack 'On Lying to Patients',* *Newsweek*, 4 June, 1979, p.13.

Strasser, Mark 'Mill and the right to remain uninformed,' *The Journal of Medicine and Philosophy*, 11, 1986, pp.265-278

Chapter Eight
Determinism and Free Will

The last theory we shall deal with is the theory of **determinism**. This states that *every event has a cause*. Strictly speaking, then, determinism is not a theory of normative ethics but the doctrine of universal causation. Its implications for ethics are so important, however, that it has been a constant focus of debate since the beginning of philosophy. The question it raises is whether human beings possess **free will**. If they do not, then they cannot be held morally responsible for their actions; and if they cannot be held morally responsible for their actions, then the business of morality becomes meaningless.

When do we consider a man morally responsible? In our earlier discussion of psychological egoism, it was suggested that, if someone is to be held morally responsible for his actions, he must at the very least be capable of performing them. We do not blame Smith for what he could not do but for what he was capable of doing but didn't. This, we remember, was the meaning of the expression 'Ought implies can.'[1] A moral situation is one in which the individual can choose a particular course of action. Conversely, a non-moral situation is one in which he either has no choice, or more frequently has that choice dictated to him by something (or someone) over which he has no control. I am not to blame if I cannot breathe under water, it being physically impossible; nor am I to blame if I cannot draw a round square, it being logically impossible. Nor am I held morally responsible if forced at gunpoint to commit a crime or if, suffering from a neurosis called pyromania, I cannot help setting fire to buildings. In these last two cases the courts recognise that I am, in a special sense, less free than the normal citizen and sentences are adjusted accordingly.

But what if it could be shown that all human actions are caused by factors outside our control? It is this question which raises the philosophical problem of determinism and free will. People certainly behave as if they are free, as if they have a series of real choices open to them, and nowhere is this more apparent than when they make moral decisions. But suppose this is not the case? Suppose that behind these choices lies a whole range of antecedent circumstances, environment, heredity, and so on, which compels us, like the pyromaniac, to act in the way we do. In that case we should have to conclude that none of us is free, that none of us is responsible for our actions, and that moral decision is an illusion. In all matters of human choice, so the argument runs, a man cannot choose to do what he ought to do but rather does what he must.

Philosophers have reacted to this problem in a variety of ways. First there are the so-called **hard determinists**, who accept determinism and therefore reject freedom and moral responsibility. Then there are the so-called **libertarians**, who accept freedom and moral responsibility and therefore reject determinism.

---

1. See above, p. 19

Common to both groups is the assumption that free will and determinism are incompatible. This assumption is, however, rejected by a third group, the so-called **soft determinists** or **compatibilists**, who argue that determinism is essential to the notion of free action. Let us now examine each of these three positions.

HARD DETERMINISM

Hard determinists maintain that everything in the universe, including all human actions and choices, has a cause which precedes it; and that this is the same as saying that once the cause has occurred the thing itself (the effect) will occur. This argument, known as the theory of universal causation, carries with it the further proposition that all events are in principle predictable. If we know the causal law according to which events of the type A are followed by events of the type B – i.e. that whenever friction occurs, heat occurs – then we can safely predict that, provided certain conditions remain constant, whenever a particular A-type event occurs (rubbing my hands) it will be followed by a particular B-type event (my hands get warm). The undoubted popularity of this argument stems from the fact that it is both a fundamental presupposition of science and a matter of common sense. Thus we light the fuse in the confident expectation that a particular event (the explosion) will occur: if it doesn't we look for an alternative explanation. We assume that something has gone wrong in the causal chain of events. Was the fuse dry? Has the bomb been tampered with? Admittedly there are many things whose causes we do not know; but even in these cases we rarely, if ever, consider these things to be uncaused. Instead we seek to discover the cause which we assume exists. So doctors will admit that there are diseases with unknown causes; but they are less likely to accept that there are diseases without causes.

The determinist case has gained in strength with the modern development of such disciplines as psychology, sociology, and anthropology. With their increasing ability to account for human feelings and emotions, the belief has grown that man himself, like everything else in the animate and inanimate world, acts in accordance with causal laws. Human beings are seen less as free agents and more as complicated bits of machinery, the workings of which are fully governed by environmental and genetic factors, and the performances of which are theoretically predictable once these factors are known. This, of course, is not to say that anyone *knows* the causal explanation for any given human choice or action: all that is being claimed is that such an explanation is theoretically possible. Our ignorance of what the particular causal law may be does not invalidate the determinist proposition that this law exists and is in principle knowable.

It follows from this, says the hard determinist, that, when a man appears to have a moral choice, this appearance is an illusion. Indeed, he argues, it is precisely because we are invariably ignorant of what causes these choices that we believe that they are uncaused in the first place. A classic case of this is suggested by the philosopher John Locke (1632-1704). Suppose that a sleeping man is placed in a locked room. On awakening he decides to stay where he is, not knowing that the room is already locked. This is a real decision taken by him, it is freely made and he might have decided to leave; but in reality he has no choice and it is only his ignorance of his true condition which made him think otherwise. So it is with our moral choices. We think we are free when we decide to do X and not Y; but in fact we are not. For these decisions are causally determined: they are the effects of previous causes, and these causes of still earlier causes, back and back. This is the reason why we cannot be held responsible for our actions.

These conclusions have important consequences. Take, for example, the role of punishment. Punishment, to be just, must presuppose moral blame; and no person can be held morally blameworthy if deprived of their freedom of choice. What, therefore, prevents an attorney from entering a plea of 'diminished responsibility' – diminished, that is, on account of the causal laws governing his client's actions – for *all* his clients, irrespective of offence? Why, for example, do we distinguish between the kleptomaniac and the thief? Surely it is because we believe that the kleptomaniac, unlike the thief, is possessed by such powerful compulsions to steal that he cannot help doing what he does. The hard determinist argues that this is unfair to the thief: we are judging him to be morally responsible through an ignorance of what motivates him to steal. But look closely enough at his antecedents, his environment and heredity, and a different picture emerges, in which the thief, like the kleptomaniac, is also the unfortunate victim of circumstance. This is the view held by the contemporary determinist, John Hospers:

> Let us suppose it were established that a man commits murder only if, sometime during the previous week, he has eaten a certain combination of foods – say tuna fish salad at a meal also including peas, mushroom soup, and blueberry pie. What if we were to track down the factors common to all murders committed in this country during the last twenty years and found this factor present in all of them, and only in them? The example is, of course, empirically absurd; but may it not be that there is some combination of factors that regularly lead to homicide? . . . When such specific factors are discovered, won't they make it clear that it is foolish and pointless, as well as immoral, to hold human beings responsible for crimes? Or, if one prefers biological to psychological factors, suppose a neurologist is called in to testify at a murder trial and produces X-ray pictures of the brain of the criminal; anyone can see, he argues, that the cella turcica was already calcified at the age of nineteen; it should be a flexible bone, enabling the gland to grow. All the defendant's disorders might have resulted from this early calcification. Now, this particular explanation may be empirically false; but who can say that no such factors, far more complex, to be sure, exist?[2]

Perhaps the most famous case in which similar determinist arguments were employed by the defence occurred in 1924. Two youths, Nathan Leopold and Richard Loeb, kidnapped and murdered a 14-year-old boy, called Bobby Franks. The two killers were wealthy and highly intelligent, being respectively the

---

2. 'What Means This Freedom?' in *Determinism and Freedom in the Age of Modern Science*, ed. Sidney Hook, New York, New York University Press, 1958.

youngest graduates of the universities of Chicago and Michigan. In order to demonstrate their contempt for society and its conventional morality, the two planned the perfect crime. Their plan went wrong, they were quickly caught, and confessed. At their trial, the death penalty was demanded. For over twelve hours in his summation to the jury, Clarence Darrow, the most celebrated American attorney of his day, pleaded for mercy:

> Nature is strong and she is pitiless. She works in her own mysterious way, and we are victims. We have not much to do with it ourselves. Nature takes this job in hand, and we play our parts. . . .
>
> What had this boy to do with it? He was not his own father; he was not his own mother; he was not his own grandparents. All this was handed to him. He did not surround himself with governesses and wealth. He did not make himself. And yet he is compelled to pay. . . .
>
> To believe that any boy is responsible for himself or his early training is an absurdity. . . . If his failing came from his heredity, I do not know where or how. None of us are bred perfect and pure; and the colour of our hair, the colour of our eyes, our stature, the weight and fineness of our brain, and everything about us could, with full knowledge, be traced with absolutely certainty to somewhere. If we had the pedigree it could be traced just the same in a boy as it could in a dog. . . .
>
> If it did not come that way, then . . . if he had been understood, if he had been trained as he should have been it would not have happened.
>
> If there is a responsibility anywhere, it is back of him; somewhere in the infinite number of his ancestors, or in his surroundings, or in both. And I submit, Your Honor, that under every principle of . . . right, and of law, he should not be made responsible for the acts of someone else.[3]

Darrow was successful in his plea: Leopold and Loeb were sentenced to life imprisonment.

Hard determinists, like Hospers and Darrow, are not saying that criminals should not be sent to prison, since evidently society must be protected from them; nor are they saying that the courts should altogether cease to blame the criminal and praise the innocent. These are, after all, devices which may cause the individual to become a different kind of person. What they do question, however, is the common assumption that criminals are morally responsible for what they do.

Morality is concerned with what people ought and ought not to do; but if what they do could not have been otherwise, if they do not possess the freedom to choose what to do, then it does not make much sense either to tell them that they ought to have done differently or to punish them for what they did. The challenge of determinism, therefore, is that it speaks of the illusion of freedom and thus of the absence of moral blame.

---

3. C Darrow, 'Attorney for the Damned,' in *Philosophy: Paradox and Discovery*, ed. Arthur J. Minton, New York, McGraw-Hill, 1976, pp.302-304.

Exercise 1

Assuming that a person should be blamed for his actions only when he has freedom of choice, in which of the following cases do you think the person involved is blameworthy? Explain your answers.

a. The soldier for saving his life by collaborating with the enemy
b. The spy for giving away secrets under torture
c. The butcher for bleeding animals to death before selling them
d. The kleptomaniac for stealing
e. The boy for stealing food when he is starving
f. The motorist for speeding to save a life
g. The motorist for speeding because he is drunk
h. The foreigner for speeding because ignorant of the speed limit
i. The husband for murdering his adulterous wife
j. The father for beating his child for cheating
k. The mother for hiding her criminal son from the police
l. The surgeon for not knowing the latest treatment
m. The linguist for failing the maths exam
n. The bank manager for handing over the money to the armed robber
o. The hypnotised woman for undressing in public
p. The drug addict for stealing from the chemist
q. The Catholic unmarried mother for having an unwanted baby
r. The Muslim, living in Manchester, for bigamy
s. The IRA activist for killing the British cabinet minister
t. The psychopath for raping the woman

LIBERTARIANISM

It would appear that if we wish to retain the idea of moral responsibility, we must reject determinism and accept that a person can, when confronted with the choice between right and wrong, act as a free agent. This view is known as **libertarianism**. This is not to say that libertarians reject determinism altogether: in general they agree that the inanimate world is mechanistic – that all events in it are mechanically caused and thus predictable – and that the mechanical chains of cause and effect may extend even to the animate world. What they deny is that the principle of universal causation applies also to *human action* and that, accordingly, human behaviour is predictable. It may well be that the kleptomaniac, left alone in a shop, will steal; but one can never be certain that he will. Physiological and psychological conditions may well dispose him towards stealing, but he may well choose to do otherwise; and in the making of this choice, says libertarianism, lies his freedom.

In presenting this argument, libertarians often distinguish between a person's formed character, or **personality**, and his or her **moral self.** Personality is an empirical concept, governed by causal laws, capable of scientific explanation and prediction, and known through observation of behaviour and psychoanalysis. The personality one has, formed by heredity and environment, limits the choices one has, and makes us more likely to choose certain kinds of actions and not others. A youth, accustomed to violence, is more likely to decide on a career of violence than someone brought up to condemn it. But however likely this may be, it is not inevitable. For if the youth is aware of the significance of his actions, it is possible that his *moral self* will counteract the tendencies of his personality and cause him to do something else: he may become a policeman instead! The moral self, therefore, is not an empirical but an ethical concept, operative when we decide what to do in situations of moral choice. Most commonly, this involves deciding between self-interest and duty, between, say, stealing and not stealing; and here the moral self is quite capable of making a *causally undetermined choice*, of subduing the inclinations of upbringing and temperament, and of deciding, through an effort of will, to do something which is not self-interested but which satisfies the sense of moral duty. In this respect, says the libertarian, the moral agent overcomes the pressures exerted upon him by his own personality and becomes morally responsible for what he does. It is this capacity that distinguishes humans from animals: the former are capable of moral choice, the latter are not. Thus C A Campbell writes:

> Here, and here alone, so far as I can see, in the act of deciding whether to put forth or withhold the moral effort required to resist temptation and rise to duty, is to be found an act which is free in the sense required for moral responsibility; an act of which the self is sole author, and of which it is true to say that 'it could be' (or, after the event, 'could have been') 'otherwise'. . . .
>
> There is X, the course which we believe we ought to follow, and Y, the course towards which we feel our desire is strongest. The freedom which we ascribe to the agent is the freedom to put forth or refrain from putting forth the moral effort required to resist the pressure of desire and to do what he thinks he ought to do. . . .
>
> . . . the very function of moral effort, as it appears to the agent engaged in the act, is to enable the self to act against the line of least resistance, against the line to which his character as so far formed strongly inclines him. But if the self is thus conscious here of combatting his formed character, he surely cannot possibly suppose that the act, although his own act, issues from his formed character? I submit, therefore, that the self knows very well indeed, from the inner standpoint, what is meant by an act which is the self's act and which nevertheless does not follow from the self's character . . . the 'nature' of the self and what we commonly call the 'character' of the self are by no means the same thing. The 'nature' of the self comprehends, but is not without remainder reducible to, its 'character'; it must, if we are to be true to the testimony of our experience of it, be taken as including also the authentic creative power of fashioning and refashioning 'character.'[4]

For the determinist, this argument is very unsatisfactory. If it is admitted that my personality may be determined by such things as heredity and environment, why is it not accepted by the libertarian that my moral attitudes may be

---

4. 'On Selfhood and Godhead,' in *Philosophy: Paradox and Discovery*, ed. Arthur Minton, New York, McGraw-Hill, 1976, pp. 342-343, 345-346.

conditioned in precisely the same way? Why is it agreed that a person is free to choose between duty and desire but not free in any other choices that he or she makes? The libertarian, in other words, has assumed the existence of free will in situations of moral choice but has provided no evidence for it.

The libertarian's reply is commonly composed of three additional arguments. In the first he makes a straightforward appeal to the facts of experience. Each of us frequently has the direct and certain experience of being a self-determining creature. We have this experience when we decide to drink tea rather than coffee, to read this book and not that, to wear a brown jacket and not a green one – and so on. This experience is common to all of us, and extends also to those whose choices are sometimes restricted (e.g. the alcoholic or drug addict). For while, within a particular range of activities, they cannot help what they do, generally speaking they still have the immediate experience of decision, of making a choice, of deciding, for example, whether or not to take the dog for a walk or whether to go to Spain for their holidays. In these areas they do not feel any special difficulty in making up their minds, and indeed are able to compare these situations with those over which they have no control. Thus, although recognizing the limits of their freedom, they still have sufficient other experiences to sustain their general belief in the existence of free will.

An appeal to the facts of experience is also involved in the libertarian's second argument. This concerns an analysis of the way in which we make our decisions: the **act of decision-making.** All of us do this at some time or other and the process can be of varying length and benefit; but that we all do this demonstrates that each of us possesses free will. This is because we can only make decisions about what to do if

a. we do not already know what we are going to do; and
b. if it is in our power to do what we are thinking of doing.

Suppose, for example, that a student is wondering whether to pay her residence fees. She may take into consideration the size of her room, the quality of her meals, and so on. Now if she decides to pay, she makes a decision: she has weighed up the pros and cons. Significantly, this would still be an act of decision even if, unknown to her, she had no money in the bank. In this case she would simply be considering what to do with money that, in her ignorance, she thought she possessed. But what she could not do is decide whether to pay or not, *knowing* that she had no money. She could not decide what action to take if she knew beforehand that only one action was open to her. Thus for someone to make a decision about something, he must believe he has a real choice, that he is capable of doing either A or B; and if he cannot do either A or B, he cannot make a choice between them. The libertarian therefore concludes that since we all do often make decisions, we must all believe that we can make choices, that we are free. In this way determinism, which rejects the existence of free will, is itself rejected by the universal experience of decision-making.

To this the determinist has a ready reply. No one disputes that people believe they are free and that this belief is supported by the experience of decision-making; but this is not to say that we actually are free. After all, a man can, on the evidence of certain experiences, believe many things – that the sun is shining, that his wife is faithful, that the world will end on Thursday; but believing these things does not mean that they are true. In the same way, the evidence of decision-making can deceive us into believing that free will exists. Benedict Spinoza (1632-1677) puts the point succinctly:

> Thus the infant believes that it is by free will that it seeks the breast; the angry boy believes that by free will he wishes vengeance; the timid man thinks it is with free will he seeks flight; the drunkard believes that by a free command of his mind he speaks the things which when sober he wishes he had left unsaid. Thus the madman, the chatterer, the boy, and others of the same kind, all believe that they speak by a free command of the mind, whilst, in truth, they have no power to restrain the impulse which they have to speak, so that experience itself, no less than reason, clearly teaches that men believe themselves to be free simply because they are conscious of their actions, knowing nothing of the causes by which they are determined.
> . . . Consequently, those who believe that, who believe that they speak, or are silent, or do anything else from a free decree of the mind, dream with their eyes open.[5]

The libertarian's third argument is designed to meet this objection, and it employs an important philosophical distinction. This is a distinction between two kinds of knowledge and, accordingly, between two kinds of truths or propositions which may be known to be true or false. Consider the following lists:

List A
All bachelors are unmarried
Black cats are black
You cannot simultaneously be in the room and out of it

List B
This table is brown
It is raining
George has one eye

The statements in List A are said to be **necessarily true**. This is because they could not possibly be false and because their truth is established independently of sense experience. So, for example, being an 'unmarried man' is precisely what is meant by the concept of 'bachelor': it is a type of proposition which is true *by definition* and which requires no empirical verification. The statements in List B are said to be **contingently true** because these are verified by sense experiences and because they may conceivably be false (given the possibility that these experiences may deceive me). So however certain I may be that George has one eye, this does not mean that he has. My own eyesight may be misleading me.

Another example will make this distinction clearer. If A, B and C are three positive numbers, and if A is greater than B, and B greater than C, then it is

5. Spinoza, *Ethic,* trans. W Hale White and revised by Amelia Hutchinson Stirling, London, T Fisher Unwin, 1894, pp.111-112.

necessarily true to say that A is greater than C. This is true by definition and its negation necessarily false. If, however, A, B and C are three runners, and A has always beaten B, and B has always beaten C, it does not follow that A must necessarily beat C. Our experience may lead us to predict that he will, but he may be wrong. On the day of the race, A may damage a tendon and lose. From this we conclude that, in our observation of the world around us, it is impossible to achieve complete knowledge; that, in the world of contingent events, the possibility of error always exists.

Exercise 2

Which of the following statements are necessarily true (or false) and which contingently true (or false)?

a. $2 + 2 = 4$
b.   2 trees + 2 trees = 4 trees
c.   A straight line is the shortest distance between two points
d.   Napoleon was Emperor of the French
e.   All men die
f.   If A knows B, and if B knows C, then A knows C
g.   If A precedes B, and if B precedes C, then A precedes C
h.   It is cold at the top of Everest
i.   No object can be red and green all over
j.   A triangle is a three-sided figure
k.   A man cannot walk on water
l.   Every man has a mother
m.   I am reading this sentence
n.   Skyscrapers are tall buildings
o.   Time moves forwards, not backwards
p.   Something exists

This distinction between necessary truth and contingent truth forms the basis for the libertarian reply to the determinist. The determinist, we remember, has argued that the evidence in support of free will – the experience of deliberation – while admissible as evidence for the *belief* in free will, is not admissible as evidence for the *existence* of free will. It is always possible, he says, that our experience may deceive us and that no such free will exists. In that case, replies the libertarian, the determinist is saying no more than that this experience, like all other experiences, belongs to the realm of contingency and is subject to error. One can say the same of the experience that I am sitting in this room or that last Thursday I got married: in either case it remains logically possible that I am hallucinating or that a clever hypnotist has been at work. The question to ask, therefore, is not whether I can be deceived by my experiences – this is now seen to be a truism – but whether the possibility of deception means that I cannot accept these experiences as *sufficient evidence for the truth of my beliefs.* For example, it is clear that I could be imagining things when I say 'I have a pen in my hand'; but does this mean that I have no good reason for saying that a pen is actually in my hand? Certainly not, says the libertarian, because the truth of this belief is justified by the immediate and direct evidence of sense experience itself. So overwhelming is this experience that I do not deny its basis in fact. Admittedly, the evidence for the pen's being there is insufficient when matched against the requirements of necessary truth, which excludes error; but it is not insufficient when matched against the requirements of contingent truth, which accepts error. For contingent truth is precisely that which is reached on the basis of corrigible evidence: it is something which, although fallible, I can still accept as being beyond reasonable doubt and view with certainty.

This, then, is the libertarian's case against the determinist. If the experience of deliberation is to be rejected as evidence for the existence of free will because this experience could deceive us, then *any evidence whatsoever*, so long as it is based on experience, must be rejected for the same reason. We must reject, for example, those experiences from which we deduce that there are material objects, that there are other minds besides our own, that there are such things as past events. We must discard, in other words, the *standard of evidence* which belongs to the realm of contingency and adopt instead a position of almost total scepticism, which few can accept and in which no valid or certain judgements can ever be reached about ourselves and our world. To put the matter more bluntly, if the act of deliberation is incompatible with the theory of determinism, and if this act must be counted among the certain facts of our experience, then this act must take priority over the theory, and the theory of determinism must be rejected.

SOFT DETERMINISM

It would seem, then, that we must choose between, on the one hand, the belief in universal causation and, on the other, the belief in the existence of free will, it being accepted by both determinists and libertarians that these two beliefs are incompatible. This incompatibility is, however, rejected by the third party to the dispute, which says that human freedom and moral responsibility, far from being incompatible with determinism, is incomprehensible without it. This is the position taken by the so-called **soft determinists** or **compatibilists**.

The assumption that determinism is inconsistent with free will is, says the soft determinist, the result of considerable confusion about what precisely we mean when we say we are free. It is certainly true that freedom is incompatible with *fatalism*, the view that human beings are powerless to change the cause of events and that 'what will be, will be'; but it is not incompatible with determinism – the theory of universal causation – *if among the choices that determine our actions we count our own choices and desires.* To clarify this point, consider the following cases:[6]

---

6. Given by W T Stace, *Religion and the Modern World*, New York, Harper & Row, 1952.

A

Gandhi fasting because he wanted to free India
Stealing bread because one is hungry
Signing a confession because one wanted to tell the truth
Leaving the office because one wanted one's lunch

B

The man fasting in the desert because there was no food
Stealing because one's employer threatened to beat one
Signing because the police beat one
Leaving because forcibly removed

Now it is clear that the actions in column A conform to what the libertarian would call free actions; and indeed, with the exception of the last example, to what he would call moral actions. These are, to use Campbell's terminology, *causally undetermined choices*, in which the person involved, through an effort of will, subdues his natural inclinations and decides for duty rather than self-interest. Thus the moral self overcomes the dictates of his personality. These actions, however, are clearly distinguishable from those in column B, which are causally determined choices. These are actions controlled by antecedent conditions, and any appearance of freedom that they might possess is, says the hard determinist, an illusion.

But is it true, asks the soft determinist, that the actions in column A are uncaused? Take the case of Gandhi. To say that 'Gandhi fasted in order to free India' is the same as saying 'Gandhi's *desire* to free India *caused* him to fast'; and this desire, we may presume, was the result of other causes, such as his previous education and upbringing, the teaching of his Hindu faith, his experiences of British rule, and so on. In other words, while the precise causal explanation of Gandhi's fast may be difficult to establish – and here the historian and psychologist will help us – it is nevertheless accepted by the soft determinist that such an explanation is theoretically possible and that, if known, it would provide us with a complete and true account of why Gandhi did what he did. The conclusion is, therefore, that the actions in group A are no less determined than those in group B, and that all human actions, whether free or not, are wholly governed by causes.

If all the events in columns A and B have causes, what is the difference between them? The difference, continues the soft determinist, lies in whether these events have *internal* or *external* causes. If you leave the country because you want a holiday, you leave of your own free will (i.e. voluntarily). If you leave because expelled by the authorities, you are forced to go (i.e. involuntarily). But in each case your action is caused. When you leave freely, the cause is your desire to go abroad; when you leave unfreely, the cause is the force exerted upon you by the government. When, therefore, the cause is internal (ie, the result of your own wishes or desires), you acted voluntarily and of your own free will; but when the cause is external (i.e. contrary to your wishes or desires) you acted involuntarily and under compulsion.

According to the soft determinist, this distinction between internal and external causes explains why freedom (and so moral responsibility) is not only compatible with determinism but actually requires it. *All* human actions are caused. Here determinism is right. For if these actions were uncaused, they would be completely unpredictable, capricious, and therefore irresponsible. Thus when we say a person acted freely, we do not mean that his action was uncaused but rather that he was not compelled to do it, that he was under no kind of 'external' pressure, that he himself chose to act in this manner. Here he acts as a free agent, even though his actions are just as much caused as those that are unfree. Similarly, when we say that a person is responsible for his actions, we still presuppose that he is a free agent; but the freedom presupposed does not deny causal antecedents but rather accepts that freedom has causes, albeit causes of a particular kind. These causes proceed from the desires, beliefs and characters of those concerned: they are, that is, the 'internal' causes and the consequence of the particular psychological condition of each individual. This freedom, then, is the ability of every human being to act in accordance with his or her own wishes; and the more we know of these wishes, the more we are able to predict what each individual would do, if not what they will do.

If determinism is compatible with freedom in this last sense – if one's wishes and desires may be counted among the causes of one's actions – then it is also compatible with moral responsibility. If X could not have acted otherwise because of some 'external' physical constraint, if Smith's inability to swim prevented him from saving the drowning child, then clearly no moral responsibility is involved and X is not to blame. But if not being responsible means that X could not have acted otherwise because of certain 'internal' constraints – that Smith did what he did because of certain wishes or desires on his part – then this is the same as saying that X was responsible. What he did was of his own doing, freely undertaken, and the result of his character; that it was precisely his being X (and not Y) that caused, and was responsible for, his action.

Questions: Determinism and Free Will

1. Give examples from your own experience to support the thesis of determinism. Can you offer any alternative interpretations of these examples?

2. 'On Darrow's argument, all crooks get off.' Discuss.

3. Is it true to say that criminals have no more control over their behaviour than the sick have over their state of health? If it is true, what are the implications for our judicial system?

4. What argument, based on the immediate experience of decision-making, is introduced by the libertarians as evidence of free-will?

5. Give examples from your own experience to support Campbell's distinction between personality and moral self. How would a hard determinist assess these examples?

6. Does soft determinism adequately overcome the problems posed by hard determinism?

7. What premise, common to both libertarians and hard determinists, is rejected by soft determinists? On what grounds do they reject it?

8. Explain the libertarian claim that hard determinists are guilty of an unscientific assessment of the nature of evidence. Do you agree?

9. Analyse the following argument: In urging us to accept their theory as true, determinists provide a disproof of that theory. For the decision whether to accept the theory or not implies free will. There is no point in urging us to accept a theory if our choice is determined anyway.

10. Read the following account by A S Neill of his school, Summerhill. Do you think the absence of rules achieves the desired effect? What rules, if any, do you think essential for the education of children?

> Summerhill began as an experimental school. It is no longer such; it is now a demonstration school, for it demonstrates that freedom works.
>
> When my first wife and I began the school, we had one main idea: to make the school fit the child – instead of making the child fit the school.
>
> I had taught in ordinary schools for many years. I knew the other way well. I knew it was all wrong. It was wrong because it was based on an adult conception of what a child should be and of how a child should learn. The other way dated from the days when psychology was still an unknown science.
>
> Well, we set out to make a school in which we should allow children freedom to be themselves. In order to do this, we had to renounce all discipline, all direction, all suggestion, all moral training, all religious instruction. We have been called brave, but it did not require courage. All it required was what we had – a complete belief in the child as a good, not an evil, being. For almost forty years, this belief in the goodness of the child has never wavered; it rather has become a final faith . . .
>
> What is Summerhill like? Well, for one thing, lessons are optional. Children can go to them or stay away from them, for years if they want to. There is a timetable, but only for the teachers.
>
> The children have classes usually according to their age, but sometimes according to their interests. We have no new methods of teaching, because we do not consider that teaching in itself matters very much. Whether a school has or has not a special method for teaching long division is of no significance, for long division is of no importance except to those who want to learn it. And the child who wants to learn long division will learn it no matter how it is taught.
>
> Children who come to Summerhill as kindergarteners attend lessons from the beginning of their stay; but pupils from other schools vow that they will never attend any beastly lessons again at any time. They play and cycle and get in people's way, but they fight shy of lessons. This sometimes goes on for months. The recovery time is proportionate to the hatred their last school gave them. Our record case was a girl from a convent. She loafed for three years. The average period of recovery from lessons aversion is three months.[7]

7. A S Neill, *Summerhill: A Radical Approach to Child Rearing,* London, Victor Gollancz, 1962, pp. 4-5.

Bibliography: Determinism and Free Will

Berofsky, Bernard (ed.) *Free Will and Determinism*, New York, Harper &
Row, 1966. A comprehensive anthology.

Campbell, C A 'On Selfhood and Godhead', *Philosophy: Paradox and Discovery*, ed Arthur J Minton, New York, McGraw-Hill, 1976.

Darrow, Clarence 'Attorney for the Damned', *Philosophy, Paradox and Discovery*, ed Arthur J Minton, New York, McGraw-Hill, 1976. An excellent
general anthology.

Dworkin, G (ed.) *Determinism, Free Will and Moral Responsibility* Englewood
Cliffs, NJ: Prentice-Hall, 1970.

Honderich, T (ed.) *Essays on Freedom of Action*, London, Routledge & Kegan
Paul, 1973.

Hospers, John 'What Means This Freedom?, *Determinism and Freedom in
the Age of Modern Science*, ed. S Hook, New York, New York University
Press, 1958. The volume contains papers given at a New York symposium.

Neill, A S *Summerhill: A radical approach to child rearing*, London, Victor
Gollancz, 1962

Pears, D F (ed.) *Freedom and the Will*, London, Macmillan, 1963.

Spinoza, Benedict de. *Ethic*, trans. W Hale White, and revised by Amelia
Hutchinson Stirling, London, T Fisher Unwin, 1894.

Stace, W T. *Religion and the Modern World*, New York, Harper & Row, 1952.

Thornton, Mark *Do we have Free Will*? Bristol, Bristol Classical Press, 1989.
Very readable introduction to the major issues.

Watson, G (ed.) *Free Will*, Oxford, Oxford University Press, 1982.

Chapter Nine
Discussion: Medical Practice and the
Ethics of Behaviour Control

According to the libertarian model of man, all human beings have the capacity to act freely, the existence of free will being a matter of immediate experiential fact. Having acted in one way the individual feels certain that he could have acted in another. Man therefore achieves intellectual and moral maturity only after a long struggle: he is responsible for his victories, for which he deserves praise, and he is responsible for his failures, for which he deserves blame. This view of human beings is, however, rejected by **behaviourism**. There are many versions of behaviourism, all of which employ the principles of determinism, but the two most important are **psychological behaviourism** and **bio-behaviourism**.

PSYCHOLOGICAL BEHAVIOURISM

The origins of psychological behaviourism are generally attributed to the opening paragraph of an essay published in 1913 by John B Watson (1878-1958), the so-called 'father' of this branch of the behavioural sciences:

> Psychology as the behaviorist views it is a purely objective experimental branch of natural science. Its theoretical goal is the prediction and control of behavior. Introspection forms no essential part of its methods, nor is the scientific value of its data dependent upon the readiness with which they lend themselves to interpretation in terms of consciousness. The behaviorist, in his efforts to get a unitary scheme of animal response, recognises no dividing line between man and brute. The behavior of man, with all its refinement and complexity, forms only a part of the behaviorist's total scheme of investigation.[1]

Watson's suggestion that behaviour can be predicted and controlled follows from the determinist doctrine of universal causation. If everything in the universe is bound to the law of cause and effect, then it is possible to predict, once a certain event X has occurred, that it will have a particular result Y. By the same token, if I can set up certain conditions such that X occurs, then I have controlled the appearance of Y. Thus Watson and his followers maintain that man operates within a wholly determined and orderly world and that all human behaviour, including man's moral decisions, are governed and controlled by causal processes which are in principle knowable. Imperfect prediction of human events and decisions is thus due to imperfect knowledge. What are regarded as free actions are no more than those actions which an embryonic science of human behaviour has not as yet explained.

Less familiar to us is Watson's rejection of what he calls 'introspection' and 'consciousness'. We are all sufficiently aware of our thoughts (or

---

1. 'Psychology as the Behaviorist Views It,' *Psychological Review*, 20 (March 1913) p. 158.

consciousness) that we can, after a process of interior analysis (or introspection) report them to others. The trouble is, says Watson, that these reports are so varied, and the thoughts they describe so private, that no reliable classification of these inner sensations is possible. For example, after a process of self-examination, X may conclude that he is in love with Y, and even tell Y that he is; but there is no means whereby an outsider, even Y, can conclusively check that X really does feel like this. Thus Watson rejects introspection as unscientific: he does not deny the existence of so-called 'mental events' but maintains that, because the evidence available cannot be observed by any one except the subject, it cannot provide the data of psychology. Some of Watson's followers go even further:

> The simplest and most satisfactory view is that thought is simply behavior – verbal or non-verbal, covert or overt. It is not some mysterious process responsible for behavior but the very behavior itself in all the complexity of its controlling relations, with respect to both man the behavior and the environment in which he lives. The concepts and methods which have emerged from the analysis of behavior, verbal or otherwise, are most appropriate to the study of what has traditionally been called the human mind.[2]

What, then, does determine the behaviour of men? Watson believed that two factors were decisive. There is *heredity*, which involves merely the inheritance of a body and certain physiological features: one does not inherit intelligence, talents, or instincts. There is also the effect of one's *environment*. By the manipulation of man's surroundings, so Watson contends, the behaviour of man can be decisively altered, and even quite complicated activities – like driving a car, solving a problem, falling in love – can be broken down into a series of learned responses. This is clear from Watson's famous remark:

> Give me a dozen healthy infants, well-formed, and my own specified world to bring them up in and I'll guarantee to take any one at random and train him to become any type of specialist I might select – doctor, lawyer, artist, merchant-chief and, yes, even beggar-man, and thief, regardless of his talents, penchants, tendencies, abilities, vocations, and race of his ancestors.[3]

The process whereby environment affects behaviour Watson called 'conditioning'. His theory of conditioning was influenced by the pioneering work of the Russian physiologist Ivan Pavlov (1849-1936). During his research into the digestive glands of dogs, Pavlov noticed that, while all dogs salivate when eating, the secretion of saliva also occurred before: it was enough for them to see the food or even hear the sound of their keeper's footsteps. In his research, Pavlov carried this to the point where his animals would react to a particular stimulus that did not normally cause salivation (i.e. the dogs would salivate on hearing a musical note played before feeding). Because food invariably causes salivation, Pavlov calls food an 'unconditional stimulus' and the salivation an 'unconditioned response'. A musical note, on the other

2. B F Skinner, *Verbal Behavior*, New York, Appleton-Century-Crofts, 1957, p.449.
3. J B Watson, *Behaviourism*, London, Kegan Paul, 1925, p.82.

hand, because it does not usually produce salivation, is called a 'conditioned stimulus'. In Pavlov's experiments, the dogs had so associated the conditioned stimulus (music) with the unconditional stimulus (food) that it produced the unconditioned response (salivation). When this occurs, says Pavlov, the unconditional response may be called a 'conditioned response'. According to him, a conditioned stimulus always results in a conditioned response.

Classical or Pavlovian conditioning, to which Watson is indebted, explains a type of learning familiar to us all. Schoolchildren, for example, associate bells with food and the beginning of lessons, while at other times such sounds may denote danger. This form of conditioning cannot however account for all human behaviour. Hungry children (or dogs) will not sit patiently all day waiting for a bell to be rung: if no food appears, they will seek it for themselves. People, in other words, are not always conditioned by their environment but will often operate on it to get what they want. Such actions are called *operant behaviours* and they are learned by *operant conditioning*

The notion of operant conditioning is associated with the work of B. F. Skinner (1904-1990), whom many regard as the foremost behaviourist of our day. What is being conditioned here is not a reflex response (like salivation) but any kind of spontaneous behaviour that the animal performs without specific stimulus. Operant conditioning therefore changes *voluntary* behaviour and thus is sometimes known as *behaviour modification*. If a rat in a 'Skinner box' accidentally hits a lever that produces food, it will eventually associate the lever with the food and press the one to get the other: it has learnt a new voluntary behaviour. The most important step in operant conditioning is to arrange the environment so that the desired behaviour occurs. To achieve this, the behaviour must be reinforced. Reinforcement that is pleasant (like rewarding or praising) Skinner calls **positive reinforcement**. For pushing the lever the rat is rewarded with food, the diligent student with high marks, the industrious worker with increased pay, and so on. **Negative reinforcement**, on the other hand, acts to remove an unpleasant stimulus, which is a reward in itself. So the rat, suffering from electric shocks, will hit the lever to switch off the current. In human affairs this same technique can be seen in the government's threat of punishment to achieve obedience – in the pain, humiliation or discomfort it may and does inflict on the individual. Reinforcement distinguishes between those things we *have* to do to avoid punishment and those we want to do for rewarding consequences. Both methods increase the probability that an action or behaviour will be repeated.

BIO-BEHAVIOURISM

The second form of conditioning is for many people the more alarming and potentially dangerous of the two. This is achieved through bio-behavioural control, otherwise known as 'genetic engineering' or **eugenics**, which seeks to maintain or improve the genetic makeup of the species. As first used by the English geneticist Francis Galton in the late 19th century, the term 'eugenics' stood for a blatantly racist and class-orientated programme, his intention being to allow the more suitable races a better chance of prevailing over the less suitable.

> It may seem monstrous that the weak should be crowded out by the strong, but it is still more monstrous that the races best fitted to play their part on the stage of life, should be crowded out by the incompetent, the ailing, and the desponding.
>
>   The time may hereafter arrive, in far distant years, when the population of the earth shall be kept as strictly within the bounds of number and suit-ability of race, as the sheep on a well-ordered moor or the plants in an orchard-house; in the meantime, let us do what we can to encourage the multiplication of the races best fitted to invent and conform to a higher and generous civilization, and not, out of a mistaken instinct of giving support to the weak, prevent the incoming of strong and hearty individuals.[4]

While subsequent eugenicists have denounced Galton's prejudices, many still share his belief that mankind is in a state of progressive genetic decline and that some form of eugenics is necessary to halt it. With Crick and Watson's discovery in 1953 of DNA (deoxyribonucleic acid) – the code which deter-mines each individual's genetic structure – this is now a genuine possibility, allowing for the direct improvement of genotypes and the reduction of genetic deficiencies through genetic surgery.

Human eugenics can be divided into two types, positive and negative. **Positive eugenics** involves the planned breeding of so-called superior men and women to improve the genetic pool and to create new inherited capacities for future generations. This parallels techniques already used successfully in agriculture for the production of new hybrid breeds of cattle and other food stuffs. The most famous example of positive eugenics is the sperm-bank proposed by Hermann J. Muller, the leading eugenicist of recent years. The sperm of selected men, chosen for their intellectual and social desirability, would be collected, frozen and stored in sperm-banks, and then used in the full-scale insemination of large numbers of women. This, Muller contends, would significantly improve the human genetic stock. Indeed, Muller goes so far as to suggest that certain specific qualities could be eugenically produced by this method: 'a genuine warmth of fellow feeling and a cooperative disposition, a depth and breadth of intellectual capacity, moral courage and integrity, an appreciation of nature and art, and an aptness of expression and of communication'.[5]

Muller's programme is not altogether far-fetched, particularly if we take into account recent developments in so-called *recombinant DNA research*. This research provides the means for freely transferring genetic information (DNA) from one cell into a cell of a different genetic background, and thus allows the gene to produce the same product regardless of the cell in which it is used. This is not cloning – which requires the transfer of all genetic material from one cell into a cell whose DNA has been removed – but it does open up the possibility of altering the genetic makeup of a test-tube embryo prior to implantation in the womb. By this means parents could decide the physical characteristics of their offspring before birth.

4. *Hereditary Genius*, London, Macmillan, 1870, p.343.
5. 'Should We Strengthen or Weaken Our Genetic Heritage?' *Daedalus*, 90 (Summer 1961) p.445.

Not surprisingly, positive eugenics has been subject to many criticisms. One is that, in making more people genetically alike, it will reduce the evolutionary advantages of genetic variation, which allows species to be more adaptable to any drastic environmental changes that may occur. Another is the notorious difficulty of fixing those characteristics considered valuable by society. We may consider intellect and beauty desirable, but there is no guarantee that our children will. Muller himself, in an early list of valuable sperm-donors, includes Marx, Lenin and Sun Yat Sen; but in subsequent lists these names are excluded and replaced by Einstein and Lincoln! But perhaps the most questionable eugenic assumption is that these desired qualities have a genetic rather than environmental basis. While it may be true that some characteristics can be genetically engineered, it is false to suppose that all can be eugenically acquired. This, indeed, is to underestimate the claims of behaviourists like Watson and Skinner, who argue that the desired characteristics are more probably controlled by environment. However strong the genetic predisposition may be to act in a certain way, it is, they argue, the effect of behavioural conditioning that is more likely to produce the desired result.

Negative eugenics is preventative genetic medicine, and I shall have more to say about it presently. Negative eugenics has the laudable objective of eliminating or treating those genes carrying disease or disability. The most widely practised example of this is *amniocentesis*, leading to therapeutic abortion. By obtaining cells from the amniotic fluid surrounding the unborn child, parents with chromosomal translocations can be told of the high risk of producing children who are mentally retarded or who possess congenital malformations. This procedure is generally regarded as a major beneficial advance in biomedical technology. Other procedures involve voluntary or involuntary sterilization.

Negative eugenics shares all the criticisms of positive eugenics, not least the problem of deciding what is genetically good and bad and the problem of deciding who makes that decision. Its major difficulty, however, is that faced by all preventative medicine: How far can the programme of prevention be extended? This appears when we move from the treatment of particular individuals (or foetuses) to the treatment of whole populations. In the particular case it may well be a clear-cut teleological judgement for doctor and parent alike that a badly handicapped child should be aborted; but to give this decision normative ethical significance – to say that foetuses with this genetic defect ought always to be aborted – is to make a further teleological judgement about the place of retarded or physically defective individuals in our society: to judge them, in other words, according to the principle of social utility. But how far can this principle be extended? Does it immediately legitimate the compulsory sterilization of retarded individuals? Does it require that marriages between people of reduced intelligence should be disallowed? Does it mandate the screening of whole populations for particular biochemical defects that can be detected in utero? And in all these questions another ethical dilemma is presupposed: the question of the invasion of privacy, and what one does with the information beyond giving it to the individuals concerned.

MEDICAL PRACTICE AND BEHAVIOURISM

Not surprisingly, psychological and bio-behavioural techniques for the control of human action directly impinge on current medical practice and have thereby given rise to a number of ethical questions of considerable public concern. Let us consider some of them.

Psychological control techniques are generally applied to those whose behaviour is, for a number of reasons, judged to do harm either to themselves or to others. In aversion therapy, for example, a modification of behaviour is sought through the application of electric shock, as in the treatment of persistent child molesters, or, as in the case of alcoholics, by the use of emetics. Many patients undergo psychological treatment voluntarily, willingly submitting themselves to programmes designed to reduce their addictions, alleviate their depressions, and correct their violent or socially unacceptable behaviour; but many do not, and in these cases patients are classified as mentally ill or mentally retarded, and involuntarily committed to mental institutions. Here they are subjected to various forms of therapy either without their consent or with consent being a precondition for their eventual release. The involuntary civil commitment of these people is justified by invoking the liberty-limiting principle of strong paternalism: that such mentally sick individuals must be prevented from doing others harm. A schizophrenic who believed in a divine voice demanding the murder of women would, on this count, be judged a serious risk to the community and so excluded from it.

This is not to say, however, that the involuntary psychological treatment of those classified as mentally ill is always justified. Two problems should be mentioned. The first has to do with the definition of 'mental illness'. Is this the name for a definable disease or a synonym for offensive behaviour? The psychiatrist Thomas S. Szasz has argued that the concept of mental illness has no cognitive usefulness, and that what defines it is not a mental disease, like syphilis of the brain, but rather a deviation from the accepted psychosocial, ethical or legal norms of the society. Mental illness thus becomes a 'problem in living', and the treatment meted out to the patient a means of dealing with deviant social behaviour.[6] In this respect, the practice of 'sane' men incarcerating their 'insane' fellow human beings may be likened to that of white men enslaving black men: it is a crime against humanity.

The second problem returns us to the question, already discussed in a previous chapter, of when paternalistic duties should outweigh autonomous rights.[7] The issue is: must free and informed consent be obtained from those whose behaviour is to be controlled? In normal circumstances one would suppose that any psychological intervention must require voluntary consent; but this is unlikely in the case of those who have been involuntarily committed, where one is very often dealing with mentally deficient persons for whom rational consent is impossible. Are we saying, therefore, that institutionalised persons forfeit their right to behavioural inviolability? The paternalistic reply is straightforward enough. Interventions to change personality are undertaken

---

6. 'The Myth of Mental Illness,' in Szasz, *Ideology and Insanity*, London & New York, Marion Boyars, 1983. See also in the same volume 'Involuntary Mental Hospitalization', pp.113-139.
7. See above, p. 126

for therapeutic purposes, that is, to benefit the patient. That the patient may be unable to appreciate where the therapeutic benefit lies, and even deny that it is a benefit, does not mean that the doctor should descend to the same level of competence and act in a way that the patient, if he had been in a more rational frame of mind, would reject as harmful to himself and dangerous to the community.

For many, however, the medical dilemmas associated with psychological behaviourism are as nothing compared to those arising from the development of bio-behavioural or genetic forms of control. On the face of it, it seems almost churlish to consider these problems at all, not least because the modern ability to detect and correct an increasing number of genetically-related disorders seems such a clear example of the laudable utilitarian ambition to reduce and eliminate suffering. But, as we shall see, moral difficulties arise when the capacity to diagnose and treat a disease is coupled with the ability to *predict* and if necessary *determine* a genetic history.

At the present time over two thousand genetic disorders have been identified. As examples we may cite Tay-Sachs disease, which is found primarily among Jewish children of Eastern European heritage, sickle-cell anaemia, a blood disorder which commonly affects blacks, cystic fibrosis, PKU (phenylketonuria), which causes retardation, and Huntington's chorea, which results in mental and physical deterioration between the ages of 35 and 50. All these are instances of *autosomal* and *recessive* genetic disease: they are autosomal because the defective genes are to be found on a pair of chromosomes that are not the sex chromosomes, and they are recessive because the disease appears only when two so-called 'heterozygous' carriers of the defective gene mate and produce an affected or 'homozygous' child. Haemophilia, because connected with mutant genes on the sex chromosomes, is an example of a recessive disease which is not autosomal. All the carriers of these recessive conditions can now be detected through genetic testing. I have already mentioned the most common of these, amniocentesis, which allows for the detection of genetic disease through analysis of the foetal cells in the amniotic fluid, and which is widely used in screening for Down syndrome. Another test which has become increasingly popular is chorionic villi sampling (CVS), a procedure performed during the first trimester of pregnancy, in which tissue is extracted from the placenta.

This ability to detect not just those who *suffer* from specific recessive traits but also those who *carry* them raises a number of important moral issues. Since most prenatal genetic analysis is undertaken with a view to selective abortion, reactions to it will largely depend on how one views abortion; on whether, for example, one accepts the foetus as a person with a moral right to life and so rights to equal protection. Many of these moral issues have been discussed already,[8] but three additional problems are worth highlighting.

The first points to a possible and deleterious change in attitude towards those human beings who are genetically defective, that is, towards those who, for one reason or another, have escaped abortion. It has been pointed out that parents who, through no fault of their own, failed to be genetically tested or who received a false prenatal diagnosis, may well feel resentful towards their offspring,

8. See above, pp. 31-32

treat them as second-class specimens and refuse permission for subsequent treatment. Quite apart from the social stigma that might now attach to them, abnormal children may also have grounds for complaint against their parents and doctors, and, as is already happening in cases of prenatal infection with syphilis and German measles, be justified in bringing legal actions against them for 'wrongful life' and to seek substantial damages for negligence where the handicap was predictable. Under these circumstances, as Kass has remarked, the 'idea of "the unwanted because abnormal child" may become a self-fulfilling prophecy, whose consequences may be worse than those of the abnormality itself.'[9]

Another issue arises from the fact that genetic testing not only identifies genetic disease but identifies those 'at risk.' If two carriers of an autosomal recessive disease have offspring, there is a 25% chance that their child will be affected, a 50% chance that it too will be a carrier, and a 25% chance that it will be totally free of the disease. This leads to the question: In situations of such high genetic risk, is reproduction immoral? Applying the utilitarian calculus, it would appear that it is. What is the net balance achieved between pleasure and pain, between avoiding harm and increasing suffering? Evidently no harm can be done to a person who does not exist nor are the rights to life of such a non-existent person being infringed. Thus just as it is not wrong to use contraception to prevent potentially healthy persons from existing, so it is not wrong to prevent potentially unhealthy persons from existing. On the other hand, the existence of such persons does increase the occurrence of actual suffering – i.e. to themselves and to their families – and does increase the risk that others will also suffer. To refrain from reproducing is thus a moral obligation placed upon those at risk: their duty is to avoid the extension of their risk to others.

Much the same conclusion can be reached from a Kantian direction. The respect that I should show to other autonomous beings rules out deliberately placing them in jeopardy: no duty of the will can therefore intentionally impose on others a risk which they have not themselves chosen to adopt. Nor can it be said that a prohibition on reproduction infringes a natural right possessed by all of us, including the bearers of genetic disease, to have families. Other options are open to us – for example, adoption, artificial insemination, *in vitro* fertilization followed by embryo implantation, egg donation and surrogate motherhood – and so to insist on exercising this right by coital means alone would be, in these special circumstances, wilful, negligent and irresponsible.

This conclusion, however, raises another difficulty. If reproduction is considered immoral in situations of genetic risk, then to what extent is coercion justified in restricting individual reproductive choices? Again, a powerful argument can be advanced in its favour. If carriers of genetic disease will not act to prevent a lethal harm being done to others, then protection must be provided by the state, particularly where the actual or potential victims lack the power and the knowledge to defend themselves, and where the voluntary cooperation of childbearing couples in preventing the transmission of disease cannot be assumed. Mandatory screening programmes should therefore be instituted,

9. 'Implications of Prenatal Diagnosis for the Human Right to Life,' in *Ethical Issues in Human Genetics*, edited by Bruce Hilton et al., Plenum, 1973, p. 190.

and coercive measures, such as compulsory sterilization or compulsory amniocentesis followed by abortion, applied to all those identified as carriers.

Screening of this kind, when taken together with the coercive measures I have mentioned, may well, if implemented, have a dramatic effect in reducing recessive genetic disease. Yet, quite apart from the financial costs of such programmes, it has been argued that the personal cost of these policies to the individual is likely to exceed any expected beneficial effects. The collection of genetic information will create a demand for its wider availability. Increasingly the right to privacy will protect no one, sensitive and hitherto confidential data will be publicly scrutinised and available to all, and those now deemed 'at risk' may well find themselves not just socially ostracised but discriminated against when seeking employment, a house, insurance or schooling.

Many of these problems are discussed in the extracts which follow. In the first Robert Neville considers the highly-charged issue of whether mildly mentally retarded persons should be involuntarily sterilised. His argument, however, is not the one normally associated with eugenics, namely, that such a policy would improve the gene pool. We should first acknowledge the real incapacities of the mentally retarded – for example, their inability to cope with pregnancy, childbirth and child rearing. Sterilization neutralises the effects of their sexual activity, and thereby enables other capacities to be realised and developed. This involuntary restriction, so Neville claims, will enhance the dignity of the mildly mentally retarded as members of the 'moral community', and allow them to participate more fully in the rights and responsibilities of membership.

The second extract is taken from an article by Joseph Fletcher. In the 1960s Fletcher achieved considerable fame as the leading exponent of so-called 'situation ethics', a moral viewpoint which was receptive to the liberal and permissive tone of the time. According to Fletcher, the most important aspect of the moral life is not a blind adherence to legalistic-deontological maxims – what he calls the *a priori* approach – but rather to the spirit of 'loving concern' which should always underpin them. This loving concern is expressed in the pragmatic and utilitarian desire to meet and fulfil human needs. Anything, therefore, that contributes to the improvement of the human lot, such as bio-behavioural control, should be enthusiastically supported.

The geneticist Marc Lappé is altogether more cautious. It is simply naive to assume that the present unprecedented acquisition of knowledge in human genetics will always serve the common good and be so easily susceptible to utilitarian equations. Lappé's main concern is with the ownership of the knowledge. The ability to look directly at a person's DNA will undoubtedly have great clinical value, enabling doctors to detect genes conferring risk of, say, Alzheimer's disease or Down's Syndrome; but at the same time questions arise about the rights of access to such information. Lappé gives many examples of the improper use and adverse consequences of genetic data, and cautions us against the facile assumption that the alleviation of suffering in one area will not increase it in another.

Extract 1: Robert Neville: Sterilizing the Mildly Mentally Retarded without Their Consent.[10]

Under certain specific circumstances it is morally permissible to sterilise some mildly mentally retarded people without their consent. At the outset of my argument I want to acknowledge that there is a grave difficulty, conceptually and empirically, in identifying which individuals belong to the relevant class of the mentally retarded. If that class is either conceptually so vague or empirically so confused that individuals who do not belong in it are inadvertently placed there, then it would be ethically impermissible to subject the class to involuntary sterilization. But let me put that difficulty aside until the end, and proceed with the argument as if we knew with acceptable exactness who the mildly retarded are and which of them meet the specified requirements for sterilization. . . .

My argument is really two arguments, one nested in the other. The first can be called the 'humble argument' for involuntary sterilization, and it attempts to make the case that involuntary sterilization is in the best interest of certain mildly mentally retarded people. The second can be called the 'philosophical argument,' and it interprets the 'humble argument' as a problem of rights and responsibilities, and attempts to show that involuntary sterilization in the right cases fosters rather than denies the membership of the mildly mentally retarded in the moral community.

The humble argument begins with certain observations. First, at least some mildly mentally retarded people are capable of engaging in and taking pleasure in heterosexual intercourse. My following remarks concern only this group; presumably those incapable of such intercourse would not need sterilization; those who, because of inexperience, do not know their capacities for pleasure should be viewed as capable of engaging in and taking pleasure from sexual activity until proved otherwise.

Second, for some mildly retarded people sexual activity is capable of being integrated into emotional aspects of affection, which can in turn contribute to positive, rewarding fulfilments of personal and social life. Freed from pregnancy, childbearing, and child rearing, an active heterosexual life can enrich the existence of some mildly mentally retarded people in much the way it can that of so-called "normals." Other things being equal, mildly mentally retarded people can benefit from and have a right to sexual activity and the social forms sexual relationships can involve, such as marriage. Capacities for marriage and long-lasting affection do not have to be clearly present, however, for the retarded to have a claim on sexual activity for purposes of pleasure alone.

Third, what begins to make the situation for the retarded 'not equal' to that for 'normals'? For mildly mentally retarded women the physiological and emotional changes that take place during pregnancy, and the violence of childbirth, are often experienced as disorientating and terrifying traumata. To the extent that a retarded man participates in the process, he too can be disorientated and lose his personal equilibrium.

Fourth, child rearing is sometimes beyond the capacities of mildly retarded people precisely because of the characteristics of their retardation. The fact that child rearing is in practice also beyond the emotional capacities of many normal people should not obscure the overwhelming difficulty that it often poses for the retarded. Now it seems a prima facie argument that children ought not to be

10. *Mental Retardation and Sterilization: A Problem of Competency and Paternalism*, ed. Ruth Macklin & Willard Gaylin, New York and London, Plenum Press, 1981, pp.181-193.

conceived if there is not some reasonable expectation that they will receive minimal care. (Note that this is not an argument that conceived children should be aborted, which is more difficult to sustain.)

Fifth, mildly mentally retarded people have a great difficulty in managing impermanent forms of contraception. I am assuming that sterilization is the only permanent contraceptive; at least it cannot be reversed without medical help. Therefore, if these mildly mentally retarded people are to engage in sexual intercourse, which is otherwise desirable, without fear of the women becoming pregnant, sterilization seems the only responsible contraceptive choice.

The humble argument, then, puts together these observations and says that the mildly mentally retarded people to whom these conditions apply should be sterilised so that they may enjoy heterosexual activity if they are so inclined. If they were not sterilised they would have to be prevented from engaging in sexual activity, or conditioned to homosexual or autoerotic sexual activity exclusively, which would be hard to guarantee. If their sex lives were not so controlled, they would run the risk of pregnancy with likely trauma for themselves and improper care for their child. If the retarded people do not or cannot give consent, then someone should have the standing to insist that the retarded be sterilised involuntarily.

An added consideration may be raised at the level of the humble argument. Who is to be sterilised, men, women, or both? The answer to that question clearly depends on the circumstances – whether the candidates are living in an institution, whether that institution is highly regulated or more informal in its management of personal associations; or, if the candidates are living outside institutions, in what kinds of settings. But generally the point of sterilization is to maximise the freedom of the mildly mentally retarded in sexual matters, and it is relevant to administer the procedure to any candidate meeting the conditions who stands to suffer harm or loss of freedom without it. . . .

My philosophical argument consists of two main parts. The first considers the objection that sterilization of the mildly mentally retarded is wrong if done involuntarily because it would thereby deny the subjects their proper place in the moral community, treating them as means only and not ends in themselves. . . . The second part raises the very large problem of who decides about sterilization in the context of the mildly mentally retarded. . . .

In that tradition of Western theory which takes most seriously the dignity of the human individual, the Kantian, one of the central concepts is that of the moral community. The dignity that should be accorded to each person as a human being consists in being regarded as a member of the moral community. Membership of that community means that a person is held to be morally responsible for his or her actions and life, and is to be held responsible by the rest of the community for assuming that responsibility. . . .

The mildly retarded suffer enough from their incapacities that special care should be taken to ensure them as full a membership in the moral community as possible. To sterilise them involuntarily, some people argue, is to do them unnecessary and dehumanising violence. It is to regard them first of all as incapable of making a responsible decision about sterilisation, thus ruling them out of membership in this respect; no defender of involuntary sterilisation could deny this fact. It is, second, to regard their sex lives and childbearing and child rearing lives as so controlled by irresponsible impulses that the people may just as well be managed like objects in those areas of life. Third, it is quite possible and indeed likely, according to this position, that sterilisation is sought for the mildly mentally retarded in order to make their custody easier, in which cases the people are treated in that respect as means only, not as ends in themselves.

In answer to these arguments let me point out three characteristics of the moral community. First, membership in the moral community is relative to the capacity for taking moral responsibility; there is no membership in the moral community under ordinary circumstances in the respects in which there is no capacity for taking responsibility. Second, most capacities for taking moral responsibility need to be developed; ordinary socialisation develops most of them. The state of moral adulthood can be defined as being in possession of the capacity to take responsibility for developing the other capacities for responsible action that may be called upon. Third, a general moral imperative for any community is that its structures and practices foster the development of the capacities for responsible behavior wherever possible, and avoid hindering that development.

The idea of a moral community is an ideal that exists in pure form only in the imagination. When the ideal is applied to actual communities, it must be tailored to the fact that some people can have only partial memberships because of limited capacity for morally responsible behavior. Children, for example, only slowly take on the capacities for full membership in the moral community, and come to be treated as full members by degrees. Ordinarily we think of young children as full human beings because of their potential to develop into adults with full capacity for responsible action; when the coherence of their lives is extended over a reasonable life span, they can be expected to have moral capacities in due season. . . .

The case of the mildly mentally retarded is somewhat different from that of children and from the limited capacity of the mentally ill or senile. Like children, their capacities for development may be far greater than would have been imagined a few years ago. But unlike children, the pacing and sequencing of their development does not lead to emotional maturity at the same time they reach bodily maturity. For instance, the emotional and intellectual capacities to manage conventional birth control methods, to adjust to pregnancy, or to raise children do not develop by the time their physical development and their social peers among nonretarded people are ready for sexual activity.

Neither, sometimes, does the capacity to make informed decisions about sterilisation. Indeed, if one were to say that heterosexual activity should be prevented among certain mildly mentally retarded people until such time as they develop the capacities for responsible behavior regarding pregnancy, or for consenting to surgical sterilisation, the result is very likely to be the prevention of heterosexual activity altogether. As the humble argument says, this approach would amount to preventing the development of an important capacity for responsible behavior in areas that would be possible if an active sex life were possible, and would therefore be contrary to the imperative that the moral community foster such capacities.

Mildly mentally retarded people are like certain kinds of mentally ill people in that, from the adult perspective, there are certain areas of life in which they may lack capacities for responsible behavior and other areas where they may have them. But they are unlike mentally ill people in an important respect. A mentally ill person is conceived to be a member of the moral community because even though a proxy might exercise some of his or her responsibilities, he or she is believed to have the structure of a person who possesses the capacities for those responsibilities. . . .

Paternalism and proxy are models for enabling persons – children and the mentally ill, respectively – to enjoy membership in the moral community when they themselves have capacities for only partial membership. Another model is needed for the limited capacity of mildly mentally retarded people, one which I propose to call the model of "involuntary restrictive conditions." The model depicts mildly mentally retarded people as members of the moral community on the condition that they meet certain restrictions. Just as people with bad eyesight may be licensed to drive with the restriction that they wear glasses, so mildly mentally retarded people may be required to meet certain restrictions in order to be members of the moral community.

The analogy with driver's licenses is imperfect, however, because a person with bad eyesight can always choose not to drive and thereby not to wear glasses. But a person cannot choose to be in or out of the moral community; one is either in the position to be held responsible or one is not. Mildly mentally retarded people, and perhaps other groups, must meet the restrictions as conditions for being in the community. Therefore, from the standpoint of mildly mentally retarded people, the restrictive conditions are involuntary. . . .

Who sets the policies regarding the treatment of the mildly mentally retarded? The answer is that the decision must come from the political process (again informed by relevant experts, and formulated by broad intellectual dialogue). The reason for locating the decision in the political process is that that is the only legitimate way by which individuals can be dealt with against their wills by due process. But there are two normative factors within the political process. One is that the process should conform to whatever political norm structures it – for instance, that of a representative democracy. According to this factor, what the political process decides about mildly mentally retarded people is legitimate if due political procedures have been followed. The other normative factor, however, is the demands of being a moral community, since the political process is the vehicle for actualising those demands. A political decision is moral if it accords with what is required as a minimum for a moral community.

If the sterilization of mildly retarded people, subject to appropriate limitations, does indeed foster important capacities for morally responsible behavior, and if a moral community ought to foster such capacities where possible, the warrant for politically deciding to sterilise certain mildly retarded people is a moral one, not merely one of political legitimacy. There is a prima facie obligation to foster people's capacity for responsibility, since this capacity is the basis of their membership in the moral community. Paradoxically, to refrain from sterilisation is to do them the violence of preventing them from participating in the moral community in one of the important respects of which they are capable. . . .

Extract 2: Joseph Fletcher: Ethical Aspects of Genetic Control[11]

The ethical question . . . is whether we can justify designed genetic changes in man, for the sake of both therapeutic and nontherapeutic benefits. We are able to carry out both negative or corrective eugenics – for example, to obviate gross chromosomal disorders – and positive or constructive eugenics – for example, to specialise an individual's genetic constitution for a special vocation. Like all other problems in ethical analysis, the morality of genetic intervention and engineering comes down to the question of means and ends, or of acts and consequences. Can we justify the goals and the methods of genetic engineering?

. . . Leaving aside technical philosophical conventions, let me suggest that when we tackle right-wrong or good-evil or desirable-undesirable questions there are fundamentally two alternative lines of approach. The first one supposes that whether any act or course of action is right or wrong depends on its consequences. The second approach supposes that our actions are right or wrong according to whether they comply with general moral principles or prefabricated rules of conduct. . . . The first

11. *New England Journal of Medicine*, 185, 1971, pp. 776-783. Reprinted in *Ethics in Medicine*, ed. S J Reiser, A J Dyck & W J Curran, Massachusetts, The MIT Press, 1977, pp.387-393.

approach is consequentialist; the second is a priori.

This is the rock-bottom issue, and it is also (I want to suggest) the definitive question in the ethical analysis of genetic control. Are we to reason from general propositions and universals to normative decisions, or are we to reason from empirical data, variable situations and human values to normative decisions? Which? One or the other.

The more commonly held ethical approach is a . . . pragmatic one – sometimes sneered at by *a priorists* and called a 'mere morality of goals'. This ethics is my own, and I believe it is implicit in the ethics of all biomedical research and development as well as in medical care. We reason from the data of each actual case or problem and then choose the course that offers an optimum or maximum of desirable consequences.

For those whom we might call situational or clinical consequentialists results are what counts, and results are good when they contribute to human well-being. On that basis the real issue ethically is whether genetic change in man will, in its foreseeable or predictable results, add to or take away from human welfare. We do not act by *a priori* categorical rules nor by dogmatic principles, such as the religious-faith proposition that genetic intervention is forbidden to human initiative or the metaphysical claim that every individual has an inalienable right to a unique genotype – presumably according to however chance and the general gene pool might happen to constitute it. For consequentialists, making decisions empirically is the problem. The question becomes, 'When would it be right, and when would it be wrong?'.

What, then, might be a situation in which constructive or positive eugenics would be justified because the good to be gained – the proportionate good – would be great enough? . . . Take cloning of humans, for example, as a form of genetic engineering. . . . There might be a need in the social order at large for one or more people specially constituted genetically to survive long periods outside bathyspheres at great marine depths, or outside space capsules at great heights. Control of a child's sex by cloning, to avoid any one of 50 sex-linked genetic diseases, or to meet a family's survival need, might be justifiable. I would vote for laboratory fertilisation from donors to give a child to an infertile pair of spouses.

It is entirely possible, given our present increasing pollution of the human gene pool through uncontrolled sexual reproduction, that we might have to replicate healthy people to compensate for the spread of genetic diseases and to elevate the plus factors available in ordinary reproduction. It could easily come about that overpopulation would force us to put a stop to general fecundity, and then, to avoid discrimination, to resort to laboratory reproduction from unidentified cell sources. If we had 'cell banks' in which the tissue of a species of wild life in danger of extinction could be stored for replication, we could do the same for the sake of endangered humans, such as the Hairy Ainu in northern Japan or certain strains of Romani gypsies.

If the greatest good of the greatest number (ie, the social good) were served by it, it would be justifiable not only to specialise the capacities of people by cloning or by constructive genetic engineering, but also to bio-engineer or bio-design para-humans or 'modified men' – as chimeras (part animal) or cyborg-androids (part prosthetes). I would vote for cloning top-grade soldiers and scientists, or for supplying them through other genetic means, if they were needed to offset an elitist or tyrannical power plot by other cloners – a truly science-fiction situation, but imaginable. I suspect I would favor making and using man-machine hybrids rather than genetically designed people for dull, unrewarding or dangerous roles needed none the less for the community's welfare – perhaps the testing of suspected pollution areas or the investigation of threatening volcanos or snow-slides.

Ours is a Promethean situation. We cannot clearly see what the promises and the dangers are. Both are there, in the biomedical potential. Much of the scare-mongering by whole-hog or *a priori* opponents of genetic control link it with tyranny. This is false and misleading. Their propaganda line supposes, for one thing, that a cloned person would be a 'carbon copy' of his single-cell parent because the genotype is repeated, as if such genetically designed individuals would have no individuating personal histories or variable environments. Personalities are not shaped alone by genotypes.

Furthermore, they presume that society will be a dictatorship and that such designed or cloned people would not be allowed to marry or reproduce from the social gene pool, nor be free to choose roles and functions other than the ones for which they had a special constitutional capability. But is this realistic? Is it not, actually, a mood or attitudinal posture rather than a rational or problematic view of the question?...The danger of tyranny is a real danger. But genetic controls do not lead to dictatorship – if there is any cause-and-effect relation between them it is the other way round – the reverse. People who appeal to *Brave New World* and *1984* and *Fahrenheit 451* forget this, that the tyranny is set up first and then genetic controls are employed. The problem of misuse is political, not biological. . . .

Needs are the moral stabilizers, not rights. The legalistic temper gives first place to rights, but the humanistic temper puts needs in the driver's seat. If human rights conflict with human needs, let needs prevail. If medical care can use genetic controls preventively to protect people from disease or deformity, or to ameliorate such things, then let so-called 'rights' to be born step aside. If research with embryos and foetal tissue is needed to give us the means to cure and prevent the tragedies of 'unique genotypes', even though it involves the sacrifice of some conspectuses, then let rights take a back seat. . . .

Owing to the work of microbiologists and embryologists we are already able to produce babies born from parents who are separated by space or even by death; women are already able to nourish and gestate other women's children; one man can 'father' thousands of children; virgin births or parthenogenesis (for that is what cloning is) are likely soon to be feasible; by genetic intervention we can shape babies, rather than only from the simple seed of our loins; artificial wombs and placentas are projected by biochemists and pharmacologists. All this means that we are going to have to change or alter our old ideas about who or what a father is, or a mother, or a family. Francis Crick, co-describer of DNA, and others are quite right to say that all this is going to destroy to some extent our traditional grounds for ethical beliefs.

Extract 3: Marc Lappé: The Limits of Genetic Inquiry[12]

We are in the midst of an unprecedented explosion of knowledge in human genetics. Researchers armed with powerful new techniques are unstripping the secrets of three and a half billion years of molecular evolution. . . . Within the next few years scientists will almost certainly have pieced together a broad map of the major gene locations on the twenty-three human chromosomes. Researchers are now able to break out whole segments of human DNA and 'store' thousands of copies of each piece in clones of genetically identical bacteria. These veritable libraries of human genetic information can be loaned (or sold) to fellow researchers for more detailed analysis. . . .

This . . . raises thorny questions about ownership of knowledge. Some of the uncovered genes will be of inestimable clinical value, allowing the early detection of biochemically based disorders. Awareness of such genes might enable clinicians to anticipate serious illness or chronic disorders and design remedial interventions accordingly. It would be ethically questionable to break with the tradition of open publication of such sequences to garner profit from their sale. Similar, but less pressing arguments apply to the large number of gene sequences that will have unknown functions and hence fall into the domain of pure research.

Other gene sequences are problematic for what they appear to foretell. A case in point could be the recently uncovered loci that seem to flag the presence of genes that predispose their carriers to manic depressive illness. Should we use the knowledge of the likely presence of such "deviant" genes to abort affected fetuses? Such a program could conceivably reduce the genetic burden brought about by the presence of these genes in the human population, but it would also potentially deprive us of great poets like Sylvia Plath or politicians like Winston Churchill, each of whom may have suffered from bipolar manic depression.

Uncovering genes that regulate human vulnerability to grave illnesses such as Huntington chorea or Alzheimer's disease could increase the incidence of suicide as well as selective abortion. Given these possibilities, and the prospect of other abuses, it is prudent to examine such consequences now as we face the rapid arrival of these eventualities: What limits, if any, should be imposed on the acquisition of such knowledge? Who should control the wealth of resulting data? How should it be used? . . .

Some techniques will allow us to determine paternity, to discover the molecular fingerprinting of a felon, or to identify kidnapped children. More ominously, related techniques could be used to establish files of persons genetically at risk for acquiring AIDS following infection with the human immunodeficiency virus (HIV), knowledge which might be used to deny passports or employment. There are obviously a plethora of uses, and none is value neutral.

Some scientists have argued that the genome mapping enterprise is essentially an engineering problem and as such is morally neutral. But consider that much contemporary research focuses on disorders with early onset. Cases in point include the genes associated with phenylketonuria (PKU), cystic fibrosis, polycystic kidney disease, sickle cell anemia, thalassemia, hemophilia B, Duchenne's muscular dystrophy, and familial retinoblastoma. Since uncovery of a genetic marker or probe for such disorders permits application in prenatal diagnosis, it is evident that moral as well as scientific considerations must attend the research.

Scientists can also argue that they have a fundamental obligation to unveil the 1,000 to 2,000 individual genes responsible for the structure of the major proteins that make up the building blocks and enzymes of the human form, without consideration of the consequences. They can reasonably insist that the good outweighs the possible abuses, and that no one can reasonably anticipate all of the potential benefits. For example, who could have predicted in the 1970s that our understanding of recombinant DNA would be an essential tool that led to the rapid progress in identifying the AIDS virus in the 1980s – or the genes that might confer susceptibility to its ravages?

Because scientific information usually precedes all but its most obvious uses, there will continue to be a struggle between those who want science to march forward without restraint and those who would monitor its direction in order to assure utility of the date acquired or to minimize its adverse consequences. . . .

How then should a tool to identify the causative gene in disease or susceptibility state candidates be developed? In what familial circumstances should related

12. *Hastings Center Report*, 17 (4) August 1987, pp. 5-10

members of an affected individual be tested? Would family members then have a right to know the resulting information? Are there entities in our society other than the affected individuals themselves that have a bona fide 'right-to-know' about such sensitive genetic data? Might not persons legitimately wish neither the collection of genetic data nor its sharing even with family members?

These dilemmas faced the team that first discovered how to test for the presence of the gene for Huntington chorea. It took group leaders Nancy Wexler of New York University and James Gusella of Harvard over six years to develop an ethically acceptable plan to assist clinicians in handling the knowledge of risk status, particularly in the instance where minors or an extended family were going to be tested. Among the major ethical dilemmas were those posed by the uncovering of new at-risk persons among relatives, or the discovery of disease status in a young child. Some of these dilemmas were abrogated by denying testing to all but competent adults and assuring the confidentiality of testing of family members where requested. . . .

This type of ethical issue – which I shall call the 'locus of control question' – can be compared to those issues generated by developing any data bank that contains sensitive personal information, e.g. those created by the advent of computer-accessible records of financial and medical information. As so starkly illustrated by the acquisition of data about AIDS, a bank of human genetic information is potentially important both to the individual from whom it was collected and to others, such as health and life insurers, employers, and health maintenance organizations or group plans designed to underwrite health care for protracted periods.

A major difference between current repositories and projected genetic data banks is that financial and, to a lesser extent, medical data collections are subject to review, modification, or challenge by the identified individual. Computerized data sets also evolve over time and reflect financial or medical vicissitudes. A poor credit rating can become a good one (albeit not readily), a medical problem can be cured, a divorcée can remarry, and so on.

In contrast, a bank of genetic information will contain what may be perceived as immutable 'facts' about a person. Except for technical errors, a genetic profile is likely to be a permanent fixture of one's biological legacy. Unlike a financial or medical catastrophe, a genetic one (say, a gene mutation for Huntington chorea) cannot usually be averted or restored. . . . In this sense, gene probing is qualitatively different from drug testing. In drug screening, a 'positive' urinary test provides only a small window for discerning deviance. When a pattern of abuse is confirmed, presumably rehabilitation is possible, with greater or lesser social or medical sequelae. But a 'positive' gene test, say, for manic depressive illness, provides an ineradicable marker of deviance with potentially lifelong social consequences to the affected individual.

From a societal perspective, a gene probe for manic depression may be seen as akin to AIDS antibody testing: in both instances, testing leads to the uncovering of a marker of varying prognostic value but substantial risk of social stigmatization. . . .

With their increasingly common application in prenatal diagnosis, DNA probes may be taken as an end to medical intervention itself. As defined by Lewis Thomas, such techniques might better be considered in the realm of 'half-way technologies' that provide an intermediate 'fix' for a condition. A gene probe for an affected fetus tells you it has found the defective gene. If you now abort the fetus, you are in effect negating the potential of the same genetic data to rescue that fetus. The identical gene sequence that can find an affected fetus can readily be modified to find the normal gene. The probe for the normal gene provides the instructions for making the gene product needed for its less fortunate mutant counterpart. With some imagination, genetic engineers have been able to use such 'normal' probes to 'reverse-engineer' the missing gene product, and to devise ways of putting that product, or instructions for its production, back into genetically deficient cells.

Such wholesome and patently useful applications of gene probes may be thwarted by their earlier – and easier – applications as simple markers of a fetus slated for abortion. This pattern may be happening in prenatal diagnosis for phenylketonuria and beta thalassemia. In both instances, DNA probes have permitted early diagnosis of affected fetuses. While abortion for PKU-positive fetuses (of which there are three variants of differing severity for this treatable disorder) has not yet been widely encouraged, the knowledge of the existence of the specific genes for such variants is currently not denied to prospective parents.

If PKU probes are allowed into widespread use as prenatal diagnostic reagents, this will turn on its head the traditional end of previous PKU screening programs: the detection and successful treatment of a genetic disease. . . .

Questions

1. What kind of society would you like to see established today? Using the techniques of bio-behaviorism, how would you set about achieving it?

2. How would you define 'mental illness'? How would you distinguish it from 'social deviancy'?

3. Should there be unlimited and unregulated use of psychological techniques on violent or dangerous offenders?

4. Do you agree that involuntary sterilization should apply to the mildly mentally retarded? Should it apply to all other groups incapable of rearing children? If so, which groups?

5. Is carrying to term a foetus with Down's Syndrome an example of parental irresponsibility?

6. 'Genetic screening is no more invasive of privacy than income tax.' Discuss.

7. Construct an argument for the mandatory use of pre-marital genetic screening.

8. What factors should a doctor bear in mind before telling a patient that he or she has Huntington's disease? Would you want to be told? Would you tell your family?

9. Should insurance companies be informed about applicants who are carriers of genetic disease?

10. Is Fletcher correct to say that developments in bio-behavioural techniques will 'destroy our traditional grounds for ethical beliefs'? Give examples.

Bibliography: Behaviourism

* denotes text extracted in main text

Beauchamp, T L (ed. with J F Childers. *Principles of Biomedical Ethics*, Oxford: Oxford University Press, 1983. An application of general ethical theories to specific medical situations.

Chodoff, Paul 'The Case for Involuntary Hospitalization of the Mentally Ill,' *The American Journal of Psychiatry*, 133, no. 5, May 1976, pp.496-501.

Cox, Harvey (ed.) *The Situation Ethics Debate*, Philadelphia, The Westminster Press, 1968.

Dworkin, Gerald 'Autonomy and Behaviour Control,' *Hastings Center Report*, 6, February 1976, pp.23-28.

Fletcher, Joseph 'Ethical Aspects of Genetic Control',* *New England Journal of Medicine*, 285, (1971) pp 776-783. Reprinted in *Ethics in Medicine*, ed. S J Reiser, A J Dyck and W J Curran, Massachusetts, The MIT Press, 1977, pp 387-393.

– *Situation Ethics*, London, SCM Press, 1966.

Galton, Francis *Hereditary Genius*, London, Macmillan, 1870.

Glover, Jonathan *What Sort of People Should There Be?*, New York, Penguin Books, 1984. An argument for the use of genetic engineering for the enhancement of desirable human characteristics.

Kass, Leon R 'Implications of Prenatal Diagnosis for the Human Right to Life,' in *Ethical Issues in Human Genetics*, edited Bruce Hilton et al., Plenum, pp. 185-199.

LaFollette, Hugh 'Licensing Parents,' *Philosophy and Public Affairs*, 9, No.2, 1980, pp.182-197. An argument in favour of state regulation of reproduction.

Lappé, Marc 'Moral Obligations and the Fallacies of Genetic Control,' *Theological Studies*, 33, September 1972, pp.411-427.

– 'The Limits of Genetic Inquiry,'* *Hastings Center Report*, 17 (4) August 1987, pp.5-10.

Lear, John *Recombinant DNA: The Untold Story*, New York, Crown Publishers, 1978. A readable but often sensational account.

Muller, Hermann J 'Should we strengthen or weaken our genetic Heritage?' *Daedalus*, 90, No 3 (Summer, 1961) pp 432-450.

Neville, Robert 'Sterilizing the Mildly Mentally Retarded without Their Consent,'* in *Mental Retardation and Sterilization*, edited Ruth Macklin and Willard Gaylin, New York, Plenum Press, 1981, pp.181-193.

Purdy, L M 'Genetic Diseases: Can Having Children be Immoral?' in *Genetics Now: Ethical Issues in Genetic Research*, edited John J. Buckley, Washington, D. C., University Press of America, 1978. A strong argument against reproduction in cases of genetic risk (eg, Huntington's chorea).

Ramsey, Paul *Fabricated Man: The Ethics of Genetic Control*, New Haven & London, Yale University Press, 1970.

Richards, John (ed.) *Recombinant DNA: Science, Ethics, and Politics*, New York & London, Academic Press, 1978.

Skinner, B F *Verbal Behavior*, New York, Appleton-Century-Crofts, 1957)

Simmons, Paul D *Birth & Death: Bioethical decision-making*, Philadelphia, The Westminster Press, 1983. A discussion of abortion, euthanasia and genetic engineering from the biblical perspective.

Singer, Peter (ed. with William Walters) *Test-tube Babies*, Oxford, Oxford University Press, 1982)

Szasz, Thomas S 'The Myth of Mental Illness,' in Szasz, *Ideology and Insanity*, London and New York, Marion Boyars, 1983, pp.12-14. An argument maintaining that mental illnesses do not exist. See also in the same volume 'Involuntary Mental Hospitalization: A Crime against Humanity,' pp. 113-139.

– *The Myth of Mental Illness*, New York, Hoeber, 1961.

Watson, John B *Behaviourism*, London, Kegan Paul, 1925.

– 'Psychology as the Behaviorist Views it', *Psychological Review*, March 1913, 20, pp 158-177.

Zilinskas, R A (ed. with B K Zimmerman) *The Gene-Splicing Wars: Reflections on the Recombinant DNA Controversy*, London, Collier Macmillan, 1986.

APPENDIX
META-ETHICS

In seeking to understand the meaning and function of ethical terms like 'good' and 'bad', meta-ethics has produced a great number of different theories. These can be usefully classified under three general headings: 1) **Ethical Naturalism** (or definism); 2) **Ethical Non-naturalism** (or intuitionism); and 3) **Ethical Non-cognitivism** (or emotivism).

ETHICAL NATURALISM

This theory holds that all ethical statements can be translated into non-ethical ones, more specifically into verifiable *factual* statements. For example, consider the difference between 'Adolf Hitler committed suicide in 1945' and 'Adolf Hitler was an evil man'. The first statement is a factual statement, the truth or falsity of which can be determined by evidence. The ethical naturalist holds, however, that the second statement is also verifiable (or falsifiable) in much the same way. We can find out whether Hitler was evil either by establishing if, in his personal behaviour, he was for example cruel, deceitful or cowardly, or by determining whether his actions had evil consequences. If we find evidence that he was like this, or that his actions did have these results, then we have verified the statement that 'Adolf Hitler was an evil man'. If the evidence points in the opposite direction, then this statement is false.

Another form of ethical naturalism reduces all ethical statements to expressions of approval or disapproval, whether personal or general. So, if I say 'Mother Teresa is good', I am not saying anything about the nature or quality of the woman herself but merely that 'I approve of Mother Teresa', or that 'The majority of people approve of Mother Teresa'. Again, these statements can be conclusively verified or falsified, this time by an estimate of my and other people's psychological response to Mother Teresa. Both are verifiable (or falsifiable) by observation of oneself or by a statistical account of whether this view is shared by others.

Of the many objections to ethical naturalism, the most obvious is that it appears to prevent us from settling, or even engaging in, any kind of moral dispute. If 'A is good' simply refers to the disposition of the speaker – that he or she approves of A – then this judgement can never be wrong (except when the person concerned has misread his own feelings); it can never be disputed by another person, since it is sufficient for me to be right that I approve of it; and it will be logically compatible with any judgement that I, or anyone else, may subsequently hold. If I now hold that 'Slavery is wrong', but tomorrow hold that 'Slavery is right', both positions will be valid in so far as they accurately describe a change in my attitude. If someone else should hold that

'Slavery is wrong', this position is also valid since it is merely the expression of his or her disapproval. Nor can the discovery of any factual evidence make my position false and the other person's true (or vice versa). Although we might both change our minds when this evidence comes to light, our original claims would still be correct as expressions of our differing attitudes at a particular moment in time.

However, the most famous objection to ethical naturalism comes from G E Moore (1873-1958). In his book *Principia Ethica*[1] Moore argues that all forms of ethical naturalism, by seeking to define moral words like 'good', 'bad' and so on in non-moral terms, commit what he calls 'the naturalistic fallacy'. His argument is based on a technique he devised for testing when proposed definitions were correct or incorrect. He called this 'the open question technique'. The word 'brother', for example, has the definition 'being male and being a sibling'. This definition makes the question, 'I know George is a brother, but is he male and a sibling?' pointless because the first part of the sentence has already supplied the answer to the question. It is what Moore calls a 'closed question': the properties denoted by the words 'male' and 'sibling' represent a necessary condition for anyone to be a brother. But if I then ask the question, 'I know George is a brother, but is he a teacher at Harvard?' this is not a senseless question since the definition of George as a brother says nothing about whether he teaches at Harvard. This is what Moore calls an 'open question': the properties denoted by the words 'teacher at Harvard' do *not* represent a necessary condition for anyone being a brother. Moore concludes that a definition is correct when the question asked is closed and incorrect when the question is open. Asking an open question, in other words, means that the two expressions being used do *not* mean the same thing.

Now, since Moore maintains that all naturalistic definitions of ethical terms will result in 'open questions', his claim is that no ethical term can be defined solely in terms of any naturalistic property. To suppose otherwise is to commit the 'naturalistic fallacy'. Thus, the proposition 'Hitler was evil' cannot be substantiated by evidence of his cruelty because I can still ask the open question, 'I grant that Hitler was cruel, but nevertheless is cruelty evil?' The legitimacy of this question means that being evil cannot be defined by the fact of cruelty. And the same can be said of the identification of 'good' with 'I approve of it'. While it would be ridiculous to ask the closed question 'I approve of it, but do I approve of it?' it would not be silly to ask the open question 'I approve of it, but is it good?' Hence the identification of good with my approval cannot be supported.

According to Moore, then, any attempt to define ethical language by means of naturalistic terms (e.g. 'good' as 'pleasure', 'happiness', 'desire', 'approval', 'virtue', 'knowledge' and so forth) is mistaken. For any theory which argues that the good life is identical with any natural property is guilty of the naturalistic fallacy, which assumes that goodness is something that can be grasped by an act of direct observation.

---

1. *Principia Ethica*, Cambridge, Cambridge University Press, 1903, pp. 5-21.

ETHICAL NON-NATURALISM

Having exposed the naturalistic fallacy inherent in all forms of ethical naturalism, Moore now proceeds to his own moral theory. This is known as *ethical_non-naturalism.*. If ethical language can never be reduced to factual statements, then, as we have seen, it can never be regarded as true or false on the basis of observable evidence. Does this mean that ethical statements can never be considered true or false? Moore denies this. We do possess another method of verification, in which we decide whether an ethical proposition is true or false through a process of *moral intuition*. Here it becomes *self-evident* to us that something is good or not. For example, if we say 'Mother Teresa is good', this statement is not verifiable by observation and experience. Yet nevertheless we say that the statement is true – and *correctly* say that it is – because we can immediately see that a property of moral goodness does belong to this woman. But what is this property? It is, says Moore, a unique and indefinable quality, something which, although it cannot be analysed, we can recognize is possessed by somebody or not. In this sense it is like the colour 'yellow': it is what Moore calls a 'simple notion', which you cannot explain to anyone who does not already know it; but, unlike 'yellow', which is a *naturalistic* quality that can be observed, 'goodness' cannot be so perceived. 'Goodness', then, is a *non-natural* property, the presence of which cannot be decided by the senses but is know intuitively none the less.

> . . . If I am asked 'What is good?' my answer is that good is good, and that is the end of the matter. Or if I am asked 'How is good to be defined?' my answer is that it cannot be defined, and that is all I have to say about it . . .
>
> 'Good', then, if we mean by it the quality which we assert to belong to a thing, when we say that the thing is good, is incapable of any definition, in the most important sense of that word. The most important sense of 'definition' is that in which a definition states what are the parts which invariably compose a certain whole; and in this sense 'good' has no definition because it is simple and has no parts. It is one of those innumerable objects of thought which are themselves incapable of definition, because they are the ultimate terms by reference to which whatever *is* capable of definition must be defined.[2]

There are many difficulties with this theory, not the least being that it appears, like ethical naturalism, to rule out the possibility of moral disagreement. If good is a non-natural property that cannot be analysed through the normal procedures of observation and investigation, then what exactly is it that Moore is claiming to *know* by intuition? This becomes difficult to establish once we realize how notoriously hard it is to decide between intuitions. If I intuit that 'The President will be assassinated tomorrow' and you intuit that he won't be, then tomorrow we can decide which of our intuitions was correct; but this, be it noted, has been decided by sense-experience and not by intuition. If, however, sense-experience is disallowed, where shall we turn to decide between our intuitions? If they contradict each other, both cannot be right; but each *will* be

---

2. *Op.cit.*, pp.6, 9-10.

right for the person whose intuition tells him so. It seems, then, that we are forever prevented from knowing which intuition is true (or false) since, on Moore's theory, the only method of verification common to intuitionism is the self-evidence of the intuition itself.[3]

ETHICAL NON-COGNITIVISM

Ethical naturalism and ethical non-naturalism are both *cognitive* theories of meta-ethics: they both maintain that ethical propositions communicate a type of *knowledge*. Ethical naturalism argues that this knowledge can be scientifically verified or falsified. Ethical non-naturalism denies this and claims instead that ethical propositions ascribe a certain indefinable quality to objects and actions and that these propositions will be deemed true or false by the process of intuition. *Ethical non-cognitivism* rejects both these positions. Naturalism is denied because, as Moore demonstrated, it commits the naturalistic fallacy; and Moore's own position is rejected because there exists no simple, unanalysable quality called 'good' disclosed by intuition; because, indeed, ethical propositions are *non-cognitive*, communicating no knowledge whatsoever and containing nothing therefore that can be rendered true or false. The statement 'George is a liar' does assert something which is either true or false; but the ethical statement 'Lying is wrong' asserts nothing at all, not even that the speaker disapproves of lying. Thus ethical statements, although they may look as if they are communicating some information, are in fact cognitively meaningless.

What, then, is the function of ethical statements according to ethical non-cognitivism? For the English philosopher, A J Ayer, in his book *Language, Truth, and Logic*,[4] their function is purely 'emotive': either to express the feelings and emotions of those who employ them – and to this extent they are more like screams, groans or grunts of pleasure – or to arouse feelings in others or to stimulate action, primarily through commands. Consider, for example, the difference between someone who says 'I am in pain' and another who says 'Ouch!' The first person is *asserting* or *describing* that he is in pain (and this assertion or description is true if he is in pain and false if he isn't). The second person is not asserting or describing anything at all. The word 'Ouch!' is merely expressing or displaying their pain, something they could equally well express by their posture, facial expression or other kind of non-verbal action. In the same way, a mother who commands her child to 'Always tell the truth' is expressing not so much her own feeling towards truthfulness but her desire to develop this particular feeling in her offspring. According to Ayer, just as one would not say that a cry of pain or a command is true or false, so it is also incorrect to say that ethical judgements, which express feelings and issue commands, are true or false. If Carol says 'Stealing is right' and Mary says 'Stealing is wrong',

3. For further criticisms of Moore's position, see G C Field, 'The Place of Definition in Ethics,' *Proceedings of the Aristotelian Society*, 32 (February, 1932) pp.79-94; and W K Frankena, 'The Naturalistic Fallacy,' *Mind*, 48 (October, 1939) pp. 464-77. Both articles are reprinted in *Readings in Ethical Theory*, ed. J Hospers and W Sellars, New York, Appleton-Century-Crofts, 1952, pp.92-102, 103-14.

4. *Language, Truth and Logic*, London, Victor Gollancz, 1936, pp.102-114. Ayer restates his position in 'On the Analysis of Moral Judgments,' which appears in his *Philosophical Essays*, London, Macmillan, 1954, pp.231-249.

this is equivalent to shouting 'Hurrah for stealing' and 'Boo to stealing'. They are expressing a feeling, a feeling of approval or disapproval; but they are not describing these feelings or even asserting that they have them (although one might be able to infer from their exclamations that they do have them). This distinguishes the theory from the theory of ethical naturalism. There, the speaker was stating a proposition which could be scientifically tested (that he or she had or had not a particular attitude); but here all that is being expressed is the feeling itself or the desire to arouse this feeling in others.

Ethical non-cognitivism does, however, share with ethical naturalism the criticism that, if ethical statements make no cognitive claims, no contradiction between conflicting claims is possible and no moral disagreement can take place. To meet this objection, a less extreme version of the non-cognitive theory has been suggested by C L Stevenson in his book *Ethics and Language*.[5] Stevenson argues that moral disagreements about what is right and wrong are possible because they very often turn out to be 'disagreements in attitude,' and that these disagreements in attitude are themselves based on 'disagreements in belief'. The point to note is that disagreements in belief *can* be resolved by evidence. For example, A may express the moral attitude that 'Drivers ought to wear seat-belts'. Let us say that A's attitude is here supported by his belief that government statistics about fatal accidents are correct. If, however, B can demonstrate that these statistics are incorrect, then it is possible that A will change his mind and withdraw his original moral claim. Here B has refuted A and changed A's attitude. Stevenson concludes that to say that the difference between A saying 'X is right' and B saying 'X is wrong' is always merely a difference in approval, and that neither can be invalidated, is incorrect. For A's approval of X may, in many instances, be founded on a belief which evidence can show is unjustified.

One final amendment of ethical non-cognitivism should be mentioned. This is the theory of *prescriptivism* proposed by R M Hare in his book *The Language of Morals*. For Hare, the primary function of the statement 'X is good' is not only to express an attitude or produce one in others but to *commend*, that is, 'to guide choices, our own or other peoples', now or in the future.'[6] Hare readily admits that this commendation or prescription of action is the non-cognitive component of ethical sentences, but such sentences also contain cognitive elements. For in commending X we are saying two things: first, that X actually possesses certain characteristics or properties that make it good; and second, that we know these characteristics are good because they conform to the standards or criteria of goodness that we commonly appeal to when we make judgements of this sort. For example, if I say 'That motor-car is a good one', I am, first, commending it as the sort of car that would be good to buy; and second, commending it because it has particular qualities that make not only it commendable but any motor-car that possesses them commendable:

---

5. *Ethics and Language*, New Haven, Yale University Press, 1943. See also Stevenson's 'The Emotive Meaning of Ethical Terms,' *Mind*, 46 (January, 1937), pp.14-31. Reprinted in Hospers and Sellars, *op.cit.*, pp. 415-429.
6. *The Language of Morals*, Oxford, The Clarendon Press, 1952, p. 126.

When I commend a motor-car I am guiding the choices of my hearer not merely in relation to that particular motor-car but in relation to motor-cars in general. What I have said to him will be of assistance whenever in the future he has to choose a motor-car or advise anyone else on the choice of a motor-car or write a general treatise on the design of motor-cars (which involves choosing what sort of motor-cars to advise other people to have made). The method whereby I give him this assistance is by making known to him a standard for judging motor-cars.

This example shows why Hare believes that ethical non-cognitivism is wrong in two important aspects:

1. Non-cognitivism does not recognize that a cognitive element is necessary for the support of moral judgements. For in saying 'X is good' reasons must be given for supposing that X contains 'good-making characteristics'; and whether it does or does not contain them can be factually established. In other words, when I say 'John is good', I am commending John as a model for imitation because I believe he possesses certain qualities, like courage and honesty; and whether I am right or wrong in this, whether he is actually courageous and honest, can be independently established.

2. Non-cognitivism fails to see that all moral judgements, far from referring to individual approval, function also as universal guides to choice: that anything else like X – having the same 'good-making characteristics' – will also be good and will be commended as such. We imply, in other words, that there are not just private reasons for asserting 'John is good' – that he is good merely because I approve of him – but that this statement also has universal application; that *any man of this type* will be deemed good and commended as such.

It is worth mentioning one further point made by Hare. If it is the case that we justify our moral judgements by some moral standards or criteria – those which decide, for instance, that courage and honesty are 'good-making characteristics' – what do we do when someone else rejects them? In that case, says Hare, we make a *decision of principle*: we appeal to those principles that have guided our choices and decisions and try to give good reasons why these principles, and not others, are the correct ones to adopt. We thus engage in an analysis of rival principles. What these principles are, and how we decide between them is the business of **normative ethics**.

Bibliography: Meta-Ethics

Ayer, A J *Language, Truth, and Logic*, London, Victor Gollancz, 1936
– 'On the Analysis of Moral Judgements,' *Philosophical Essays*, London: Macmillan, 1954)
Ewing, A C *The Definition of Good*, London, Routledge & Kegan Paul, 1947. Preliminary study of meta-ethics.

Foot, Philippa (ed.) *Theories of Ethics*, Oxford, Oxford University Press, 1967. An important collection of essays by Stevenson and Frankena (on Moore), Ormson and Mabbott (on Mill), Rawls and J J C Smart.

Frankena, William K *Perspectives on Morality*, ed K E Goodpaster, Notre Dame & London, University of Notre Dame Press, 1976. Includes Frankena's important essays on Moore.

Hancock, Roger N *Twentieth Century Ethics*, New York & London, Columbia University Press, 1974. Useful introductory sections on Moore, Ross, Ayer, Hare and Rawls.

Hare, R M *The Language of Morals*, Oxford, The Clarendon Press, 1962.

Hospers, John & Sellars, W (eds.) *Readings in Ethical Theory*, New York, Appleton-Century-Crofts, 1952. An extensive collection of texts, containing the important criticisms of Moore by G C Field and W K Frankena.

Hudson, W D *Modern Moral Philosophy*, London, Macmillan, 1970. Excellent introduction to meta-ethics.

McGrath, Patrick *The Nature of Moral Judgements*, London, Sheed & Ward, 1967) Contains separate chapters on Ayer, Stevenson and Hare. Moore, G. E. *Principia Ethics*, Cambridge, Cambridge University Press, 1903.

Olthuis, James H *Facts, Values and Ethics*, Assen, the Netherlands, Koninklijke Van Gorcum, 1968. Critique of Moore and the movements that followed him.

Stevenson, C L *Ethics and Language*, New Haven, Yale University Press, 1943
– 'The Emotive Meaning of Ethical Terms,' *Mind*, XLVl, January 1937) pp 14-31. Reprinted in Sellars and Hospers, *op. cit*, pp. 415-429.

Toulmin, Stephen E *The Place of Reason in Ethics*, Cambridge, Cambridge University Press, 1950. Close to the emotive theory but laying greater emphasis on the cognitive content of moral judgements.

Warnock, Mary *Ethics since 1900*, London, Oxford University Press, 1960. Chapters 1-4 contain useful short accounts of Moore, intuitionism and emotivism.

Index